THE ESSENTIAL
FERTILITY LOG

Other books by Suzanne Schlosberg

THE ESSENTIAL FERTILITY LOG

An Organizer and Record-Keeper to
Help You Get Pregnant

SUZANNE SCHLOSBERG

Da Capo
LIFE
LONG

A Member of the Perseus Books Group

Designed by Trish Wilkinson
Set in 12-point Goudy by the Perseus Books Group

Library of Congress Cataloging-in-Publication Data

Schlosberg, Suzanne.
    The essential fertility log : an organizer and record-keeper to help you
get pregnant / Suzanne Schlosberg. — 1st Da Capo Press ed. 2007.
        p.   cm.
    Includes bibliographical references.
    ISBN-13: 978-0-7382-1084-1 (pbk. : alk. paper)
    ISBN-10: 0-7382-1084-6 (pbk. : alk. paper) 1. Natural family
planning—Calendar method 2. Preconception care. 3. Records. I.
Title.
RG136.5.S35 2007
613.9'434—dc22   2006033383

First Da Capo Press edition 2007

Published by Da Capo Press
A Member of the Perseus Books Group
www.dacapopress.com

Da Capo Press books are available at special discounts for
bulk purchases in the U.S. by corporations, institutions, and other
organizations. For more information, please contact the
Special Markets Department at the Perseus Books Group,
11 Cambridge Center, Cambridge, MA 02142, or call (800) 255-1514
or (617) 252-5298, or e-mail special.markets@perseusbooks.com.

1 2 3 4 5 6 7 8 9

To Teri Breuer, for her perseverance
To Sarah Bowen Shea, for her optimism (and her TiVo)
To my husband, Paul, for his love
To my parents, for their support

EXPERT REVIEWERS

John Hesla, M.D.
Reproductive Endocrinologist
Portland Center for Reproductive Medicine
Portland, Oregon
www.portlandivf.net

Andrea Speck-Zulak, R.N.C.
Clinical Nurse Manager
Portland Center for Reproductive Medicine
Portland, Oregon
www.portlandivf.net

IMPORTANT CONTACTS

OB/GYN: _____

    NAME OF PRACTICE: _____ WEB SITE: _____

    PHONE: _____ E-MAIL: _____

    ADDRESS: _____

    NURSE AND/OR ASSOCIATE: _____

REPRODUCTIVE ENDOCRINOLOGIST: _____

    NAME OF PRACTICE: _____ WEB SITE: _____

    PHONE: _____ E-MAIL: _____

    ADDRESS: _____

    NURSE AND/OR ASSOCIATE: _____

OTHER SPECIALIST: _____

    NAME OF PRACTICE: _____ WEB SITE: _____

    PHONE: _____ E-MAIL: _____

    ADDRESS: _____

    NURSE AND/OR ASSOCIATE: _____

ACUPUNCTURIST: _____

    NAME OF PRACTICE: _____ WEB SITE: _____

    PHONE: _____ E-MAIL: _____

    ADDRESS: _____

THERAPIST OR MIND/BODY GROUP CONTACT: _____

    NAME OF PRACTICE: _____ WEB SITE: _____

    PHONE: _____ E-MAIL: _____

    ADDRESS: _____

    OTHER CONTACTS IN GROUP: _____

LAB: _____

    CONTACTS: _____ WEB SITE: _____

    PHONE: _____ E-MAIL: _____

    ADDRESS: _____

PHARMACY: _____

    CONTACTS: _____ WEB SITE: _____

    PHONE: _____ E-MAIL: _____

    ADDRESS: _____

INSURANCE COMPANY: _____ ID #_____

    CONTACTS: _____ WEB SITE: _____

    PHONE: _____ E-MAIL: _____

    ADDRESS: _____

CONTENTS

INTRODUCTION

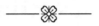

So, you're trying to get pregnant. Welcome to the club!

Chances are, your membership will be blissfully short-lived. If you're like most people, the procreation process will go something like this: Pinpoint ovulation, get it on with darling husband, break out home pregnancy test, order adorable Capri pants from Gap Maternity. If you're in your twenties, your chance of conceiving within one year runs from 86 percent to 97 percent! In your thirties, the chances are from 65 percent to 72 percent. The odds are solidly on your side.

And yet there's always that chance that your conception experience might proceed more along these lines: Read *Us Weekly* while darling husband produces sperm in plastic cup; assume the insemination position; schedule appointment with reproductive endocrinologist; store fertility drugs in fridge next to nonfat yogurt; peruse online donor-egg database featuring "cheerful law student, enjoys snowboarding."

This last scenario? That's me, more or less.

After eighteen months, lots of scheduled sex, four intra-uterine inseminations (IUIs), and two cancelled IVF cycles, I've learned this much: There's more than one way to make a baby.

I've also found that it pays to be proactive—to monitor your monthly cycle closely, to do research online, to ask your doctor and your friends plenty of questions, and to develop contingency plans and coping strategies in case your dream scenario doesn't materialize.

It's highly likely that you'll get pregnant without much rigamarole. But it's also possible that "Please provide semen sample at 8:00 A.M." will become part of your procreation process. Either way—whether you're a Fertile Myrtle or a bit of a tough nut—you're likely to get knocked up faster if you're healthy, relaxed, and well-informed about how your body operates.

That's where this book comes in handy. Think of it as your portable fertility headquarters, one central place to track all the particulars—details about your cycle, signs of ovulation or pregnancy, test results and appointments, medication protocols, workouts and relaxation exercises, thoughts and feelings. Keep the log on your nightstand, toss it in your purse when you visit the doctor or acupuncturist, or whip it out for reference when you search the Internet. Before long, your notes will reveal patterns and clues about your body that could save you months, maybe years, of frustration. What's more, the log will encourage you to stay active and to eat well, to unwind and to be kind to yourself, to remember what, and whom, you're grateful for in life.

The details you track here will prove especially useful if you end up seeking help from an ob/gyn, a reproductive endocrinologist, a fertility acupuncturist, or some other health-care professional. Chances are, you'll be asked more questions than a witness on *Law & Order:* How long is your cycle? Do you know whether you ovulate? Do you bleed after you have ovulated? How heavy is your flow and what color is it? How often do you have sex and when? Instead of relying on your memory, you can flip open your log and say, "Well, as a matter of fact . . . "

Your doctor will thank you. "If women come in prepared, we can put their treatment plan together in a short period of time, and we don't end up talking in hypotheticals," says Mark Leondires, the medical director of Reproductive Medicine Associates of Connecticut in Norwalk. "We're happier and they're happier, and hopefully they'll get pregnant sooner." Your notes and charts could point to a simple solution; for example, maybe you need to adjust the timing of your sex. Or your history may hint at a condition—inadequate hormone levels, ovulation problems, a uterine polyp—that could be confirmed by tests and corrected with medication or surgery. Or perhaps your difficulties are compounded by stress and you'd benefit from joining a mind/body infertility program.

No doubt about it, taking meticulous notes can minimize the detective work you and your doctor must do. But all this record keeping can have some unexpected benefits, too, especially if you're undergoing high-tech fertility treatments that involve complex drug regimens. "Sometimes you feel like you're spinning out of control," says Liza Charlesworth, the author of *The Couple's Guide to In Vitro Fertilization*, who went through two rounds of invitro fertilization (IVF) before conceiving twin boys. "There's something about tracking this process on hard copy—seeing all the details on paper—that makes it feel less daunting."

This book does not offer medical advice or serve as a primer on how to get pregnant. The "Recommended Books and Web Sites" section on page 167 lists several resources to supplement the information you get from your health-care professionals. *The Essential Fertility Log* is simply a tool to help you navigate this exciting and sometimes bewildering process—in short, to help you stay organized and stay sane.

THIS BOOK IS FOR YOU IF . . .

This log is designed for anyone who is trying to conceive (TTC), whether you tossed aside your diaphragm yesterday or you're in the throes of an IVF protocol. The format is flexible enough to adapt to any stage of the TTC process. You'll find this book useful if:

You've Just Started Trying to Conceive

If you've spent years trying to *avoid* pregnancy, you may not know when, or whether, you ovulate. You may have no idea when your cervical mucus starts to resemble an egg white—or why this even matters. Your log will introduce you to your body's rhythms so that you know when you're most fertile. Also, keep in mind that preconception is a critical time for good nutrition and physical activity. If you're significantly over-weight or underweight, you're more prone to hormonal imbal-ances that make it harder to conceive. Your log can help you achieve goals such as cutting back on junk food or showing up twice a week at your spinning class. The diary will serve as an important record, too, if you ultimately seek help from a doctor. Nobody expects to end up with fertility drugs in the refrigera-tor, but it's wise to think ahead.

You're Undergoing Basic Fertility Testing or Treatment

If you haven't conceived within a year—or six months, if you're thirty-five or older—don't waste time: Get thee to a doctor (ideally, a reproductive endocrinologist) ASAP. Once you've taken the plunge, there's a whole new set of data to track, including his-and-hers tests with catchy names like hysterosalpingogram and hysteroscopy (for you) and sperm motility and morphology (for him). You can use the log to record IUI cycles, Clomid or injectable medications, ultrasound results, and so on. Sure, your doctor will keep detailed records in your burgeoning file, but getting your hands on this classified dossier in a timely manner may require something like CIA-level security clearance. If the babycenter.com preconception bulletin board is discussing FSH levels *tonight*, you'll want your own data at the ready. At this stage, daily reminders to relax will do you good. It's easy to become so consumed with your treatment that you forget you have a life to enjoy.

You're Undergoing Assisted Reproductive Technology (ART)

Once you've joined the big leagues—IVF and other assisted reproductive technology (ART)—you've got more minutiae to keep track of than the editors of the *ESPN Baseball Encyclopedia*. Well, almost. Your day might look like this: three shots, four pills, an ultrasound, a blood test, an acupuncture appointment, and a phone conversation with a nurse who turns your life upside down based on the morning's test results. You need your log more than ever! Your doctor will hand you a photocopied sheet that has the protocol mapped out, but you'll need more space than those minicalendars typically provide. Besides, there's more to record than drug dosages and follicle sizes, namely, your starring role in the daily drama that is IVF. Some days you feel jazzed and in awe of the researchers who developed this marvelous technology; other days, when your butt is bruised from progesterone shots, you wish all pregnant women would spontaneously combust, along with their embroidered maternity peasant tops. You need those daily reminders to practice yoga, meditate, and read *People*.

FINAL THOUGHTS

The focus of this log, of course, is on you, but keeping track of this stuff can also be a gift to the girlfriends who will come to you with questions months or years from now. They may ask whether you found an ovulation kit useful or how you felt after your acupuncture appointments. I have four friends who tried IVF before I did, but when I'd ask them specific questions—Did you feel any side-effects from the drugs? Were you able to exercise after the egg retrieval?—inevitably they'd answer, "I can't remember! Now that I have my baby, it's all a blur." Do your friends a favor: Take notes!

With luck, this log also will end up as a gift to yourself down the line. Not long after Liza Charlesworth delivered her twins, she requested her files from her fertility doctor—a thick stack of lab results and follicle counts and ultrasound reports. "It was me—right there in black and white," says Charlesworth, who keeps the file tucked away in her office. "It's like a keepsake, a little treasure to look back on."

It is my hope that this log will serve as a keepsake for you after playing a helpful role in the arrival of your new baby.

Suzanne Schlosberg, 2006
Suzanne@suzanneschlosberg.com

MINIMIZING STRESS

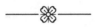

Fact: Fertility problems can do to marriages what tornadoes do to hay barns in Kansas. One of my friends—a sweet, thoughtful psychology major—spiraled so far downward during her fertility treatment that one day she yelled obscenities at her cleaning lady for failing to dust under the blender, then locked herself in a closet and huddled on the floor sobbing for two hours; the outburst prompted her normally mild-mannered husband to refer to her, not quietly, as "the second coming of Kathy Bates in *Misery*."

I mention this because it helps explain this log's emphasis on tracking emotions and stress. You'll find a journaling exercise, a daily section for recording relaxation techniques, and other charts and boxes totally unrelated to your ovulation patterns or follicle sizes. If you're new to this trying to conceive (TTC) business, you may want to disregard these sections, or maybe doodle in them. But if the process is getting you down, whether you have a common case of the blues or a diagnosis of clinical depression, filling in these blanks may give you a lift.

When it comes to getting pregnant, minimizing stress is no small matter. Studies indicate that women who are highly stressed and depressed are less likely to conceive, either naturally or via assisted reproductive technology (ART). "You get stressed because you can't conceive, which makes you more stressed, which makes it even harder to conceive," says psychologist Alice Domar, a leader in mind/body infertility research, and the director of the Domar Center for Complementary Healthcare, affiliated with Boston IVF, one of the country's top fertility centers. Some research suggests depression can cut in-vitro fertilization (IVF) success rates in half.

Scientists aren't sure why depression makes women less fertile; perhaps chemical changes in the body compromise egg quality, delay the release of eggs, or alter hormone levels. But this much is clear: When depressed women learn to manage their stress through yoga, meditation, and other mind-body strategies described in Domar's book, they're more likely to get pregnant. One study followed 184 women who'd been trying to conceive for one to two years. The results were compelling: Of the women who completed a ten-session mind-body program, 55 percent conceived, compared with 20 percent of women who received no intervention. What's more, in a follow-up study, the women in the mind/body group were significantly less depressed six months later than the women in the control group. "When you're less anxious, depressed and angry, you can make treatment decisions more clearly," Domar notes.

Research suggests that journaling—even fifteen minutes a day for four days—also is a useful tool for easing stress and even improving physical health. "You come up with tremendous insight that wells up from deep within you," says Leslee Kagan, codirector of the infertility program at the Harvard Mind/Body Medical Institute. "Usually some 'Aha!' comes to people on day three or four. It's a very freeing experience." See page 153 for details on how to do the journaling exercise.

You can also use your log to maintain what Kagan calls an "appreciation journal," a daily list of what in life you're grateful for. Research has found that counting your blessings—literally—can make you feel more optimistic and better about life as a whole, and can even reduce physical ailments. "If you're in a negative space and start to hold in your heart things you appreciate, you spiral up into positivity," Kagan says. Indeed, despite repeated setbacks, I've found it's hard to brood for too long, especially when I think of my sweet, red-headed husband, my supportive family, and my traffic-free, smog-free, hair-frizz-free life in sunny Central Oregon.

Be aware that stress can creep up on you gradually. You can keep a handle on your anxiety level, and perhaps avoid falling into a funk, by making daily or weekly notes in your log. "This way you can look back over several weeks and uncover patterns of anxiety or depression," says Domar. Use the information to sign up for yoga classes or therapy sessions or to plan downtime after a pregnancy test. "Be careful about what you schedule in life around the time you're going to find out if you're pregnant," Domar says. If you're feeling vulnerable, this may not be the time to visit a pregnant friend with three kids and a propensity for saying, "All my husband has to do is *look* at me and I get knocked up!"

Throughout the TTC process, be sure to chronicle your happy times and positive feelings as well. "When you're having a good day, write down your coping skills—all the things that work for you," Domar suggests. Maybe a massage relaxed you or chatting with an old friend perked you up; maybe you felt more cheerful after you and your husband took a long bike ride together or watched a romantic-comedy movie marathon. Later, if you're feeling down, you can refer back to this list for mood-boosting ideas.

SETTING GOALS
FOR THE
NEXT SIX MONTHS

How obvious can you get? Your goal is to get pregnant! True enough, but keep in mind that conceiving is not necessarily within your control. While you're waiting for that positive pregnancy test, consider what else you'd like to accomplish that *is* within your power, such as improving your fitness or your eating habits or your conversational Spanish. Don't put the rest of your life on hold!

When you're charting signs of ovulation or undergoing fertility treatments, it's easy to get bogged down in the day-to-day details of your cycle. It's also tempting to set aside your other aspirations—to tell yourself, "I'll start eating better when I get pregnant" or "What's the point of starting a rock-climbing class? I'm going to be pregnant soon." *Now* is the time to start working toward these goals. Who knows when you're going to conceive? Besides, once you have a bigger family, you might not even have time to master the basics of belaying and rappelling.

Use the inside cover of this book to keep sight of the big picture, and glance at it frequently to keep yourself on track. Here are some tips to help you fill out the goals page.

BACKUP GOAL

Think of a goal that you want to reach in the next six months that has nothing whatsoever to do with getting pregnant. Make it something substantial that you can work toward and feel a sense of accomplishment about, whether it's writing a screenplay, improving your tennis game, mastering Thai cooking, or earning your real-estate license. Best-case scenario, you become a pregnant realtor; worst case, you've increased your earning power.

PREGNANCY PLAN B

At every stage in your quest to conceive, it's a good idea to have a contingency plan. For example, if you're thirty-six and just starting out, Plan B might be to see a reproductive endocrinologist if you're not pregnant within six months. If you're on your second intra-uterine insemination (IUI) cycle, your plan may be to try IVF after your fourth IUI. "Don't put all your eggs in one basket, so to speak," says Alice Domar, coauthor of *Conquering Infertility*. Ask your doctor to help you choose an appropriate Plan B. This way, if your current approach or treatment doesn't pan out, you can look forward to an alternative strategy.

"Writing down Plan B made me feel like I had some control over my destiny," says Naree Viner, an executive recruiter in Los Angeles who has had one successful IVF and one unsuccessful cycle. "When you feel as if you have options, you don't get mired in disappointment."

FITNESS GOALS

If you don't already work out regularly, now is the ideal time to pick up the habit. If you're currently active, choosing new goals can help you reach the next level of fitness. Either way, you'll set yourself up for a long, healthy life—not to mention a fit pregnancy.

Research shows that women who are fit when they conceive and continue aerobic exercise throughout pregnancy tend to gain less weight and experience shorter, less complicated labors than inactive women. Studies also indicate that women who start exercising *after* conceiving need to work out more to achieve the same benefits as women who are already fit when they conceive. "You'll really be ahead of the game if you get in shape before you get pregnant," says Liz Neporent, a New York City fitness consultant who unexpectedly conceived for the first time when she was forty-four.

Identify a six-month exercise goal, and make it specific. For example, rather than write "Get fit for my pregnancy," aim to work out four days a week or sign up for a charity ten-kilometer run. If you happen to become pregnant before the event, terrific—you can walk instead of jog. If you're IVF-bound and know your workouts will be limited while your ovaries are jacked up on drugs, aim to crank up your routine before your shots begin, then to walk forty-five minutes a day during the protocol, with your doctor's permission, of course. Avoid thinking, "Well, I'm just going to be pregnant soon and I'll get fat anyway, so what's the point?"

NUTRITION GOALS

Preconception is the ideal time to improve your eating habits. This does *not* mean you should go on a diet; restrictive eating not only backfires but also can rob your body of many nutrients necessary for sustaining a healthy pregnancy. However, if you need to lose weight or your eating habits could use some improvement, it's a good idea to start making changes now. The first few months of pregnancy are crucial for your baby's development, and since you can't predict your date of conception, it's important that you prepare your body.

Your nutrition goals, like your exercise goals, should be specific, such as "Eat fruit with breakfast and a veggie with lunch" or "Switch from soda to sparkling water." If you're a caffeine guzzler, cut back to one cup of coffee a day, an amount unlikely to affect fertility. For advice on preconception nutrition, consult a registered dietitian (you can find one in your area through www.eatright.org) or read Elizabeth Somer's *Nutrition for a Healthy Pregnancy: The Complete Guide to Eating Before, During, and After Your Pregnancy*.

RELAXATION GOALS

"Relaxation goal" might seem like an oxymoron; isn't goal-setting the kind of pursuit that's pretty much the opposite of mellowing out? Nevertheless, trying to get pregnant can be stressful in countless ways, even if you've been at it for just a few months. Before you know it, "Honey, you have a great butt" becomes "Get your butt over here—my ovulation dipstick just went off." The anxiety tends to mount when your sex life is supervised by a reproductive endocrinologist and your vacations are nixed by her bills.

In some women, research suggests, stress can exacerbate infertility, so remind yourself from the get-go to stay relaxed. If you're still in the procreation honeymoon stage, your six-month goal may simply be to check in with yourself and your partner monthly to make sure you're still in good spirits and communicating well. If you are dealing with infertility and your travails are making you stressed or depressed, your goal could be to join a mind/body support group, see an infertility counselor, or try the stress-reduction techniques mentioned on page 27.

USING YOUR LOG

Rule number one for using this log: There are no rules. How much information you track and which sections you use will depend largely on your personality and where you are in your quest to conceive. If you're a writer or note taker by nature, you'll probably scribble all over the pages; if you're the type of person who'd rather code a Web site than write a sentence, your log might be pretty spare. Likewise, if you're just starting out, you might track little more than signs of ovulation and daily workouts. If you're deep into an IVF protocol, you'll probably max out the Tests/Meds/Procedures and Notes boxes.

Rule number two: No matter how many, or how few, notes you make, be sure to write things down as they happen—not three hours, or three days, later. Record your meds right after you swallow them, your period when you get it, your test results while you're on the phone with the nurse. "When people document things in real time, it's much more valid," says Mark Leondires, a reproductive endocrinologist in Norwalk, Connecticut. "Our memories are not as good as we think they are."

This section explains how to use each part of your log. No doubt, you'll come up with additional tracking methods and your own shorthand. It's your log—use it however you wish!

GOALS FOR THE WEEK

Every Monday, choose one or two key goals for the week. Whether these goals relate to exercise, nutrition, relaxation, or some other pursuit, make them concrete—for example: "Walk 45 min./day" or "Meditate 20 min./day before work" or "Make appt. with RE." To help keep your life in balance, you may want to set a goal that has nothing to do with conceiving, such as calling a friend you haven't spoken to in ages or completing a photo album you've been putting off. Be realistic when you set goals. The "Week in Review" section will hold you accountable, prompting you to note whether or not you met your goals.

PRECONCEPTION SUPPLEMENT

Check this box when you take your daily preconception/prenatal vitamin and mineral supplement. The main reason for taking these supplements is to ingest enough folic acid, a B-vitamin that's crucial early in pregnancy for preventing birth defects, such as spina bifida. You can't predict when you'll conceive, nor can you assume that you're getting enough folic acid from your diet; for these reasons, health experts recommend that TTCers consume at least 400 micrograms of folic acid daily. Most prenatal supplements contain 800 micrograms of folic acid. Ask your doctor to recommend a brand.

CYCLE DAY

Day 1 is the first day that your bleeding is red; brown spotting doesn't count. Filling in this box can help you identify patterns in your cycle. For example, if you consistently start your period on Day 29, and Day 28 always corresponds with notes such as "Breasts are throbbing" and "Snapped at Starbucks barista for putting excess foam in my latte," that's a pretty clear sign of premenstrual syndrome (PMS, which itself is a big clue that you ovulate regularly). Also, you can refer back to this box when doctors and nurses ask, as they inevitably do, "What was the first day of your last menstrual period?"

OVULATION/PREGNANCY SIGNS

Here you record what's happening with your cycle, including signs of ovulation (when an ovary releases an egg into the fallopian tube) or pregnancy.

Knowing when—or if—you ovulate is critical, not only for timing sex but also for determining whether you'll need some type of fertility treatment. If you ovulate, your odds for conceiving are best if you have sex at least once or twice within forty-eight hours of the day that you expect the egg to pop out of its follicle. Sperm can live for up to five days in fertile cervical mucus, but eggs survive only for about twelve to twenty-four hours once they're released, so it's better if the sperm are awaiting the egg than vice versa.

Keep in mind that if you're having sex two to three days a week, you needn't—and shouldn't—try to time it with ovulation. Nothing kills a good time or boosts anxiety so much as sex on demand, and the resulting stress can delay ovulation and thus cause your well-laid plans to backfire. However, if you're having sex less frequently, you do need to pay attention to the timing.

Ovulation typically happens about fourteen days before your next period—not smack in the middle of your cycle, as is commonly believed. Ovulation day varies tremendously from woman to woman and, often, from month to month. Monitoring your cycle for three months should give you a good snapshot of your body's ovulatory patterns. Here's a rundown of various ways to track ovulation, along with other items you might want to record in this box.

Your Period

Note when your period starts, how many days it lasts, whether it's painful, how heavy your flow is, what color it is, whether you have any bleeding between cycles, and whether you experience PMS symptoms such as cramping, breast tenderness, irritability, or weeping when you watch commercials on the Lifetime television channel. "All of that is helpful to know," says Larry Werlin, a reproductive endocrinologist and the medical director of Coastal Fertility Medical Center in Irvine, California. "If woman tells me she has PMS symptoms, I tell her that's a good thing. Women who don't ovulate don't have PMS."

If you're not menstruating at all, you're probably not ovulating. However, for various reasons, some women who don't ovulate do experience bleeding. Recording these clues can help you and your doctor distinguish between a real period and one that doesn't involve ovulation. Scant, irregular, really short, or symptom-free periods may suggest that you're not ovulating.

On the other hand, mid-cycle bleeding or heavy bleeding that lasts longer than a normal period could signify a uterine polyp, a hormonal problem, or some other condition that needs attention.

If you see an acupuncturist who specializes in fertility, be prepared for a friendly interrogation about your period. Says Liz Richards, a Portland, Oregon, acupuncturist: "I want to know: What color is the blood? Is it bright red? Dark red? Purple? Brown? I also ask if there's any clotting and how big the clots are. Are they the size of a pinky-finger nail or as big as a strawberry?" Richards suggests tracking the severity of menstrual cramping on a scale from 1 to 10. "All of these things help me decide what acupuncture points to use," she says.

Cervical Mucus

One relatively reliable way to assess when you're ovulating is to track the color and consistency of that goop known as cervical mucus.

Two or three days before you ovulate, the glands near your cervix release thin, stretchy, clear, plentiful mucus. This slippery stuff has the critical job of filtering out bacteria and second-rate sperm so that the good swimmers thrive during their journey to the uterus. On the days of the month when your mucus isn't slimy, it's hostile even to the Michael Phelps of sperm.

For details on how to evaluate your cervical mucus, read *Taking Charge of Your Fertility* by Toni Weschler, who describes this fluid with an enthusiasm unmatched in fertility literature. As Weschler puts it, right after your period, you experience dryness, then sticky fluid "like the paste you used in elementary school," and then you hit the "creamy" and "lotion-like" stage. The most fertile cervical fluid, she says, resembles raw egg white.

If your mucus doesn't pass through these stages, you may not be ovulating; but there may be other explanations, which your doctor can assess. For example, because the popular fertility drug Clomid can dry up cervical fluid, women on Clomid typically also undergo intra-uterine insemination (IUI), a procedure that bypasses the mucus problem by inserting the sperm directly into the uterus. Your cervical mucus may also be affected by your age. In your early twenties, you may have four or five days of fertile mucus; by your mid-thirties, you may be down to a day or two.

Ovulation Predictor Kits

Perhaps the most reliable way for most women to pinpoint ovulation is to use an ovulation predictor kit. These are available in packs of seven at any supermarket and cost from $20 to $35.

Several days before you suspect that you'll ovulate, you start peeing on a dipstick once a day. A darkened test stripe indicates that you've had your surge of luteinizing hormone (LH), which triggers ovulation by causing the follicle wall to weaken. Ovulation typically occurs from thirty-six to forty hours after the beginning of the LH surge. Doctors recommend having sex the same day as your surge, as well as a day or two later.

Ovulation predictor kits aren't 100 percent reliable. Occasionally women have an LH surge but the egg doesn't pop out of the follicle, and women with polycystic ovarian syndrome may produce false LH surges. Also, women with very long or irregular cycles may find ovulation predictor kits less useful; they'll need more dipsticks, which can get expensive.

Morning Temperature

Fallacy alert! Tracking your morning temperature, a.k.a. your basal body temperature (BBT), is *not* a useful way to time sex, yet this misconception is remarkably prevalent. Even the television crime drama *CSI* featured an episode in which one of the investigators found a BBT thermometer at a crime scene and noted that using the device "maximizes your chance of conception." It's true that hormonal changes cause your body temperature to spike about half a degree after you ovulate. However, by the time you detect this spike, you've *already ovulated*, at which point it's too late for the egg to be fertilized. That ship has sailed!

So what's the point of tracking your temperature? If you do it for a few months, your BBT patterns can help detect whether you ovulate. If your temperature doesn't change throughout your cycle, or if the numbers seem to spike and drop at random, this may be a hint—although not proof—that you're not ovulating.

You also can use your morning temperature to determine the length of your luteal phase, the portion of your cycle between ovulation and the first day of your period. Typically this phase lasts about fourteen days; but if it's shorter than ten or eleven days, you may be at risk for early miscarriage. A luteal-phase defect, as it's called, can usually be corrected easily with medication. You can track your luteal phase by counting the number of days between your rise in BBT and the first day of your period.

BBT also can be helpful in distinguishing between a late period and an early miscarriage, and for projecting how long a given cycle will be. *Taking Charge of Your Fertility* discusses at great length how to track your morning temperature and why you'd want to do it. What the book doesn't mention is that many women find the practice tedious and that there are much less labor-intensive ways to determine whether you're ovulating.

If you're interested in tracking your BBT, use the charts explained on page 141 instead of trying to track patterns in the daily log pages.

Abdominal Discomfort

Another clue that you're ovulating is an achy or painful sensation on either side of your abdomen, known as mittelschmerz, a nifty German word that means "middle pain." Only about 20 percent of women feel this discomfort or pain, so it's certainly not a reliable indicator of ovulation, but it's still worth noting in your log.

Sex

In one way, sex is like exercise: Many people don't do it as often as they think they do. Tracking how often you're having sex may not be the most romantic endeavor (and you might not want to mention this bit of note taking to your partner), but it could offer a simple explanation for why you're not getting pregnant.

Sometimes the problem isn't how often you're having sex but *when*. "Some people say they're having sex two to three times a week, but it's really two to three times on the weekend," says Mark Leondires, a physician specializing infertility. Of course, if you're not ovulating that weekend, even a record-setting sex-fest won't help.

If your husband isn't regularly ejaculating, you may want to note that, too. "I don't need to know the gory details, but if those things are written down for us, that's helpful," Leondires says.

Sexual dysfunction could indicate stress or depression, which can lead to lower sperm counts and more sexual dysfunction.

Also make a note if you have pain with intercourse, which may suggest endometriosis or damaged fallopian tubes.

Pregnancy Symptoms

Is your period late? Do your breasts hurt? Are you wiped out for no apparent reason? These are signs that you could be pregnant, and they're certainly worth noting in your log. Some women experience pregnancy symptoms within a week of conceiving; others have no indication they're pregnant for several weeks.

Just keep in mind that each of these symptoms also could mean something besides pregnancy. You can have a late period because of stress, travel, hormonal problems, or substantial weight gain or weight loss. Swollen or tender breasts could signify PMS. Fatigue can have countless explanations, anything from the flu to depression to staying up late to watch Conan O'Brien.

TESTS/MEDS/PROCEDURES

Use this space to remind yourself about upcoming acupuncture or doctor's appointments as well as to record the results of ultrasounds, inseminations, and other procedures. (There's also a chart on page 149 to record test results for you and your partner.)

If you're following an IVF protocol, this is a great place to double check that you've taken all your pills and shots and to note dosage changes during your daily conversation with a nurse. "Write down exactly what the nurses say right away," advises Liza

Charlesworth, the author of *The Couple's Guide to In Vitro Fertilization*. "You'd be surprised how quickly numbers can get confused when they're not committed to paper. It's possible you could take the wrong amount and it could blow your cycle."

EXERCISE

Exercising regularly is one of the best favors you can do for yourself while you're trying to conceive. Working out helps relieve stress and depression and control weight—important matters when you're TTC. If you're fit when you do get pregnant, you'll be better prepared to maintain a workout routine while you're knocked up; if you stick with exercise throughout your pregnancy, you'll likely gain less weight, experience fewer aches and pains, have an easier labor, and bounce back more quickly after delivery than women who were inactive. Go break a sweat!

If you haven't worked out in a while, start slowly and gradually build up to forty-five minutes or more on most days. Spend the first five to ten minutes of your workout warming up, and be sure to cool down afterward; don't sprint straight from Level 10 on the elliptical trainer to the shower. Consider hiring a certified trainer for a few sessions to get you up and running with a program.

Use this space to record physical activity, whether you're hiking, cycling, swimming, doing step aerobics, or lifting weights. Be as specific as the space allows—for example, "Jog 30 min. treadmill, 5.5." If you like tracking your workouts in more detail—for instance, listing how much weight you lifted for each strength machine—use the "Notes" box.

If you're doing an IVF cycle and have twenty follicles growing in your stimulated ovaries, your doctor probably will prohibit you from exercising, other than walking, for two to four weeks. This doesn't mean you should park yourself on the couch for a month watching the Food Channel! You can still take a daily stroll through your neighborhood.

If you're already a serious exerciser, especially a competitive athlete, the notes you make about exercise could provide your doctor with clues about your fertility. For example, excessive exercise and leanness can cause a short luteal phase, and can even cause you to stop ovulating.

RELAXATION

If you're spending oodles of money on fertility treatments, you should know that one the best investments you can make on the TTC front is free: twenty minutes a day of relaxation. "No one is too busy for relaxation," says Alice Domar. "It's actually a time saver because you waste a ton of time when you're anxious. You won't be running around looking for your keys, and you'll sleep better. There are lots of ways you get the time back."

Different techniques work for different people. You might derive a sense of calm from meditation or yoga or from a technique called mindfulness, which uses mental images—a tranquil forest, a field of poppies—to help you appreciate the here and now. Another effective technique is body scan: You breathe deeply while doing a mental scan of your entire body, releasing tension region by region.

You can learn these techniques from Domar's book, *Conquering Infertility*, or in classes held at fertility centers, hospitals, yoga centers, women's health centers, and community colleges. All these techniques have one thing in common: They activate the "relaxation response," our innate ability to ease internal stress. Triggering the relaxation response causes a decrease in your heart rate, breathing rate, muscle tension, even blood pressure and stress hormone levels. Not only will these techniques make you feel calmer the day you do them, Domar says, but they will have a carryover effect. "It's like exercise—you feel great right after you work out, but if you exercise over the course of a couple of weeks, you feel even better."

Use this space to record the technique you used on a given day, along with how you felt before and afterward. If possible, practice relaxation at roughly the same time every day so that it becomes a habit; do it twice a day if you're particularly stressed out.

Watching television or kicking back with your iPod won't trigger the relaxation response, but these types of activities are still helpful for relaxation in a nonclinical sense. If you're undergoing fertility treatments but practicing relaxation techniques isn't your bag, use the "Relaxation" space simply to jot down something enjoyable you did for yourself that day. (This is important even if you are practicing relaxation.) When your daily schedule revolves around getting poked and prodded with ultrasound wands and 25-gauge 1.5-inch needles, it's important to cut yourself some slack—to buy a cute new pair of earrings, to curl up on the couch at Starbucks with the Sunday *New York Times*, or to do whatever feels to you like a treat. It's especially important to indulge yourself after a failed fertility protocol, or even a natural cycle during which you were hoping to get pregnant.

NOTES

There are countless ways to use this space. It's a handy place to make a note of travel, illnesses, or stressful events in your life, all of which can affect ovulation. If you're doing IVF, you may need this box to supplement the "Meds/Tests/Procedures" section. Your list of drugs and tests will be quite long!

Alternately, you can use the box to express your thoughts and emotions—maybe about the TTC process, or about your relationship with your partner, your family, and your friends. Since stress and depression can affect your partner and his fertility, you might also want to make observations about his emotional state. An honest assessment of your emotions and your partner's may help your doctor guide your treatment.

The "Notes" box is also a good place to maintain an "appreciation journal," a tool that can help fertility patients who are struggling with stress and depression. Leslee Kagan, codirector of the infertility program at the Harvard Mind/Body Medical Institute, recommends that each day her patients write down three things that they appreciate. "A patient might write about appreciating her lovely garden or how the sun lights up all the different colors of her husband's beard or the support of a good friend," Kagan says. Many patients feel the appreciation journal has made them happier and closer to their husbands. "People feel it's turned things around for them," she says. "It's very connecting. They're not in a hostility mode anymore. When you move into appreciation, you move out of depression."

Even if you're not particularly stressed out, you may want to try this exercise for a week because it could help buffer you against a future bout with depression.

WEEK IN REVIEW

You may be jotting your daily notes in a hurry, between commuting home from work and whipping up dinner, or between your Lupron shot and your Doxycycline pill. So take a ten-minute breather, assess the week that has just passed, and think about the week ahead, particularly what you want to repeat or do differently. On Sunday, you may want to flip ahead to Monday and set your goals for the coming week.

Goal Check. It's common to set goals and then lose track of them. This section keeps you honest, nudging you to consider whether you met the goals you set at the beginning of the week. If you didn't, speculate why and think about what you can do differently next week to accomplish your new goals.

Total Exercise Days. Note how many days during the week you did some physical activity. This will help you monitor whether you're being consistent. Unless your doctor has instructed you otherwise, aim for at least thirty to forty-five minutes of activity a day. This needn't be a four-mile run; you could walk for twenty minutes at lunch and twenty minutes after dinner.

Total Relaxation Days. It's just as important to get into the relaxation habit as the exercise habit. If you're stressed out but find that you're practicing relaxation techniques only once a week, this space will serve as a reminder to you to make a bigger effort.

Thoughts and Feelings. Here's your opportunity to reflect on the week—whether you're in a good place emotionally, how you're getting along with your husband or partner, whether your sex life is satisfying, whether you're happy with your medical care, and so on.

SAMPLE LOG PAGES

Following are three examples of how the log might be used. These samples may give you some ideas for adapting the log to your own situation.

Sample #1. This woman is detecting ovulation with two methods—an ovulation kit and cervical mucus monitoring—and she's timing sex to coincide with the day before and day of ovulation. She's mindful that timed intercourse can be stressful on a relationship and has made notes about how she felt about the sex. She's also aiming to lose weight by exercising and boosting her fiber intake so that she feels more full on fewer calories.

Sample #2. This woman is taking Clomid, a fertility drug commonly used to induce ovulation, in preparation for an intrauterine insemination (IUI). It's early in her cycle, shortly after her period has ended, so she has no notable cervical mucus. She has been feeling stressed and is using acupuncture, Pilates, and swimming to relax. She's also working to limit her caffeine and sugar intake.

Sample #3. This woman, an IVF patient, is a few days away from her egg retrieval. She's on a complex drug regimen and undergoing frequent ultrasound and blood tests. She has noted that the dose of one of her drugs, Follistim, has been reduced. Though she's prohibited from strenuous exercise because her ovaries are enlarged, she has continued to take daily walks. She's practicing two stress-reduction techniques: mindfulness and journaling.

SAMPLE #1

WEEK

1

DATES: _July 6 - 12_
GOALS: _gym - cardio 4x_
weights 2x
nutrition - at least 10g
fiber for breakfast every day

Monday

_7 / 6_

CYCLE DAY [12] PRENATAL SUPPLEMENT ✓

OVULATION / PREGNANCY SIGNS

7 a.m. - ov dipstick
positive!
mucus, clear
and slippery

TESTS / MEDS / PROCEDURES

EXERCISE

awesome spin
class w/Jenny
- really worked

RELAXATION

NOTES

breakfast:
Kashi Go Lean - 8g fiber
strawberries - 38
_⟶ 11g_
sex with Tom! he slipped
out of work for a nooner -
quick but fun ☺

Tuesday

_7 / 7_

CYCLE DAY [13] PRENATAL SUPPLEMENT ✓

OVULATION / PREGNANCY SIGNS

mucus slippery

TESTS / MEDS / PROCEDURES

EXERCISE

15 min. elliptical
Wt. circuit 3x
abs w/ball

RELAXATION

NOTES

breakfast:
whole-wheat toast - 4g
peanut butter - 2g
banana - 3g ⟶ 9g

sex again! Not as good
as yesterday - a bit forced
but still fun

SAMPLE #2

WEEK
1

DATES: _Oct. 21- 27_
GOALS: _Pilates 2x_
swim 2x
cut back on sweets and
caffeine

Monday

10|21 CYCLE DAY 6 PRENATAL SUPPLEMENT ✓

OVULATION / PREGNANCY SIGNS

TESTS / MEDS / PROCEDURES
100 mg Clomid
- feel fine, no
symptoms

EXERCISE
Pilates mat class
w/Sara
getting stronger!

RELAXATION
zoned out for 20 min.
after class in
"quiet area"
- loved it!

NOTES
decaf vanilla latte -
no whip (160 cals)
instead of frap.
w/whip (430)
⟶ saved 270 cals

Tuesday

10|22 CYCLE DAY 7 PRENATAL SUPPLEMENT ✓

OVULATION / PREGNANCY SIGNS

TESTS / MEDS / PROCEDURES
acupuncture appt.
_8 a.m._

100 mg Clomid

EXERCISE
swam 45 min.
2000 yds.
inc. 8 x 50 sprints

RELAXATION
last 15 min. of
swimming was
really relaxing,
meditative

NOTES
felt calm after acu.
- tense when needles
went in but then
relaxed

apple and peanut butter
instead of candy bar for snack

SAMPLE #3

DATES: _Feb. 2 - 8_
GOALS: _stay relaxed for retrieval_
- and be kind to myself!
- keep walking w/pedometer
until retrieval (unless don't feel well)

Monday   2/2

CYCLE DAY 16   PRENATAL SUPPLEMENT ✓

OVULATION / PREGNANCY SIGNS

TESTS / MEDS / PROCEDURES
*ultrasound - 8:30 a.m.
aspirin, Dexameth.
Menopur - 9:15 a.m.
Follistim - 9 p.m.
Lupron

EXERCISE
walked 9,367
steps

RELAXATION
practiced mindfulness
during my walk

NOTES
doc said follicles
"look great"
12 on rt / 9 on left
biggest are 18 mm
v. excited!
*reduce Follistim to 150

Tuesday   2/3

CYCLE DAY 17   PRENATAL SUPPLEMENT ✓

OVULATION / PREGNANCY SIGNS

TESTS / MEDS / PROCEDURES
aspirin, Dexa
Menopur 9:10 a.m.

HCG 10:30 p.m.

EXERCISE
walked downtown
and back
~ 2 mi. - feel
good, not too bloated

RELAXATION
journaled for
20 min.

NOTES
trigger shot tonight
10:30 p.m. sharp!

husband's motto: "Hey
it doesn't hurt me!"
(didn't hurt me too
much either)

DAILY LOG

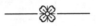

WEEK 1

DATES: _____

GOALS: _____

_____

_____

_____

Monday

___/___

CYCLE DAY [ ]   PRENATAL SUPPLEMENT [ ]

OVULATION / PREGNANCY SIGNS

TESTS / MEDS / PROCEDURES

_____

_____

_____

_____

_____

EXERCISE

_____

_____

_____

NOTES

RELAXATION

_____

_____

_____

_____

Tuesday

___/___

CYCLE DAY [ ]   PRENATAL SUPPLEMENT [ ]

OVULATION / PREGNANCY SIGNS

TESTS / MEDS / PROCEDURES

_____

_____

_____

_____

_____

EXERCISE

_____

_____

_____

NOTES

RELAXATION

_____

_____

_____

BY THE NUMBERS **1 to 2 million:** The number of eggs in the ovaries of newborn girls. **300,000 to 400,000:** Number of eggs in teenage girls. **25,000:** Typical number of eggs remaining at age 37, though the count can vary widely from woman to woman.

Wednesday ___/___

CYCLE DAY ☐   PRENATAL SUPPLEMENT ☐

OVULATION / PREGNANCY SIGNS

TESTS / MEDS / PROCEDURES

_____
_____
_____
_____
_____

EXERCISE

_____
_____
_____

NOTES

RELAXATION

_____
_____
_____

Thursday ___/___

CYCLE DAY ☐   PRENATAL SUPPLEMENT ☐

OVULATION / PREGNANCY SIGNS

TESTS / MEDS / PROCEDURES

_____
_____
_____
_____
_____

EXERCISE

_____
_____
_____

NOTES

RELAXATION

_____
_____
_____

CONCEPTION WONDERS There have been at least fifty reported cases of identical quadruplets, created when a second round of splitting occurs after a fertilized egg has already split into two embryos. The odds of this happening are about 1 in 11 million.

Friday __/__

CYCLE DAY ☐ PRENATAL SUPPLEMENT ☐

OVULATION / PREGNANCY SIGNS

TESTS / MEDS / PROCEDURES

_____
_____
_____
_____
_____

EXERCISE

_____
_____
_____

RELAXATION

_____
_____
_____

NOTES

Saturday __/__

CYCLE DAY ☐ PRENATAL SUPPLEMENT ☐

OVULATION / PREGNANCY SIGNS

TESTS / MEDS / PROCEDURES

_____
_____
_____
_____
_____

EXERCISE

_____
_____
_____

RELAXATION

_____
_____
_____

NOTES

THROUGH THE AGES In the seventeenth century, many doctors believed sperm heads contained miniature, fully formed people called homunculi, who would develop into a baby when deposited in the womb. A popular competing theory: Minihumans were housed in the egg, and sperm would trigger their growth.

Sunday

___/___

CYCLE DAY ☐   PRENATAL SUPPLEMENT ☐

OVULATION / PREGNANCY SIGNS

TESTS / MEDS / PROCEDURES

_____
_____
_____
_____
_____

EXERCISE

_____
_____
_____
_____

NOTES

RELAXATION

_____
_____
_____
_____

Week in Review

GOAL CHECK _____

TOTAL EXERCISE SESSIONS _____

TOTAL RELAXATION SESSIONS_____

THOUGHTS AND FEELINGS

2

DATES: _____

GOALS: _____

_____

_____

_____

Monday   __/__

CYCLE DAY ☐   PRENATAL SUPPLEMENT ☐

OVULATION / PREGNANCY SIGNS

TESTS / MEDS / PROCEDURES

_____

_____

_____

_____

_____

EXERCISE

_____

_____

_____

RELAXATION

_____

_____

_____

NOTES

Tuesday   __/__

CYCLE DAY ☐   PRENATAL SUPPLEMENT ☐

OVULATION / PREGNANCY SIGNS

TESTS / MEDS / PROCEDURES

_____

_____

_____

_____

_____

EXERCISE

_____

_____

_____

RELAXATION

_____

_____

_____

NOTES

BY THE NUMBERS **21.4:** Average age of first-time mothers in the United States in 1970. **25.2:** Average age of first-time U.S. moms today. **27.7:** Average age of first-time mothers in Canada. **29.4:** Average age of first-time mothers in France. **30.4:** Average age of first-time moms in Italy.

Wednesday __/__

CYCLE DAY ☐   PRENATAL SUPPLEMENT ☐

OVULATION / PREGNANCY SIGNS

TESTS / MEDS / PROCEDURES

EXERCISE

RELAXATION

NOTES

Thursday __/__

CYCLE DAY ☐   PRENATAL SUPPLEMENT ☐

OVULATION / PREGNANCY SIGNS

TESTS / MEDS / PROCEDURES

EXERCISE

RELAXATION

NOTES

MYTH VS. REALITY   **Myth:** Long-term use of the birth control pill compromises fertility and can be risky for the baby. **Reality:** It's perfectly safe to get pregnant the month that you go off the pill, and birth control pills neither accelerate nor slow down the biological clock.

Friday   __/__

CYCLE DAY ☐   PRENATAL SUPPLEMENT ☐

OVULATION / PREGNANCY SIGNS

TESTS / MEDS / PROCEDURES

EXERCISE

RELAXATION

NOTES

Saturday   __/__

CYCLE DAY ☐   PRENATAL SUPPLEMENT ☐

OVULATION / PREGNANCY SIGNS

TESTS / MEDS / PROCEDURES

EXERCISE

RELAXATION

NOTES

THROUGH THE AGES   The first home pregnancy test hit the market in 1978 and was wildly popular, but its inventors, researchers at the National Institutes of Health, were not allowed to profit from their discovery. At the time, the NIH denied its scientists royalties for discoveries made using public funds, a policy since reversed.

Sunday   __/__   CYCLE [ ]   PRENATAL [ ]
                                         DAY   SUPPLEMENT

OVULATION / PREGNANCY SIGNS	TESTS / MEDS / PROCEDURES

EXERCISE

_____

_____

_____

RELAXATION

_____

_____

_____

NOTES

Week in Review

GOAL CHECK _____

TOTAL EXERCISE SESSIONS _____

TOTAL RELAXATION SESSIONS _____

THOUGHTS AND FEELINGS

WEEK

3

DATES: _____

GOALS: _____

_____

_____

_____

Monday

__/__

CYCLE DAY [ ]   PRENATAL SUPPLEMENT [ ]

OVULATION / PREGNANCY SIGNS

TESTS / MEDS / PROCEDURES

_____

_____

_____

_____

EXERCISE

_____

_____

_____

RELAXATION

_____

_____

_____

NOTES

Tuesday

__/__

CYCLE DAY [ ]   PRENATAL SUPPLEMENT [ ]

OVULATION / PREGNANCY SIGNS

TESTS / MEDS / PROCEDURES

_____

_____

_____

_____

EXERCISE

_____

_____

_____

RELAXATION

_____

_____

_____

NOTES

BY THE NUMBERS **1954:** First successful birth from frozen sperm. **1984:** First baby born from a frozen embryo. **1996:** First successful birth using frozen eggs. **2000:** Birth of first babies—twins—conceived from both frozen eggs and frozen sperm. **2005:** First baby born using a frozen donor egg from a commercial egg bank.

Wednesday ___/___

CYCLE DAY ☐   PRENATAL SUPPLEMENT ☐

OVULATION / PREGNANCY SIGNS

TESTS / MEDS / PROCEDURES

EXERCISE

RELAXATION

NOTES

Thursday ___/___

CYCLE DAY ☐   PRENATAL SUPPLEMENT ☐

OVULATION / PREGNANCY SIGNS

TESTS / MEDS / PROCEDURES

EXERCISE

RELAXATION

NOTES

CONCEPTION WONDERS   A sperm head measures 1/4,000 of an inch in diameter, and an egg is about 1/200 of an inch. Yet using microscopic tools, embryologists can inject a single sperm into an egg, enabling men with extremely low sperm counts to father their own genetic children.

Friday   __/__

CYCLE DAY ☐   PRENATAL SUPPLEMENT ☐

OVULATION / PREGNANCY SIGNS

TESTS / MEDS / PROCEDURES

_____
_____
_____
_____
_____

EXERCISE

_____
_____
_____

RELAXATION

_____
_____
_____

NOTES

Saturday   __/__

CYCLE DAY ☐   PRENATAL SUPPLEMENT ☐

OVULATION / PREGNANCY SIGNS

TESTS / MEDS / PROCEDURES

_____
_____
_____
_____
_____

EXERCISE

_____
_____
_____

RELAXATION

_____
_____
_____

NOTES

THROUGH THE AGES   An Egyptian papyrus circa 1350 BCE describes a pregnancy test in which a woman urinated on wheat and barley seeds. If the barley grew, it meant she was carrying a boy; if the wheat grew, a girl. A 1963 investigation found this test to be 70 percent accurate, likely because of the elevated estrogen levels in pregnant women's urine.

Sunday

__/__

CYCLE DAY ☐   PRENATAL SUPPLEMENT ☐

OVULATION / PREGNANCY SIGNS

TESTS / MEDS / PROCEDURES

EXERCISE

RELAXATION

NOTES

Week in Review

GOAL CHECK _____

TOTAL EXERCISE SESSIONS _____

TOTAL RELAXATION SESSIONS _____

THOUGHTS AND FEELINGS

WEEK
4

DATES: _____

GOALS: _____

_____

_____

_____

Monday
___/___

CYCLE DAY ☐   PRENATAL SUPPLEMENT ☐

OVULATION / PREGNANCY SIGNS

TESTS / MEDS / PROCEDURES
_____
_____
_____
_____

EXERCISE
_____
_____
_____

RELAXATION
_____
_____
_____

NOTES

Tuesday
___/___

CYCLE DAY ☐   PRENATAL SUPPLEMENT ☐

OVULATION / PREGNANCY SIGNS

TESTS / MEDS / PROCEDURES
_____
_____
_____
_____

EXERCISE
_____
_____
_____

RELAXATION
_____
_____
_____

NOTES

BY THE NUMBERS   **20 to 25:** Percent chance of conceiving in a given month for women in their early twenties. **15 to 20:** Percent chance in late twenties and early thirties. **10:** Percent chance in early thirties. **8:** Percent chance from middle to late thirties.

Wednesday   __/__

CYCLE DAY ☐   PRENATAL SUPPLEMENT ☐

OVULATION / PREGNANCY SIGNS

TESTS / MEDS / PROCEDURES

EXERCISE

RELAXATION

NOTES

Thursday   __/__

CYCLE DAY ☐   PRENATAL SUPPLEMENT ☐

OVULATION / PREGNANCY SIGNS

TESTS / MEDS / PROCEDURES

EXERCISE

RELAXATION

NOTES

MYTH VS. REALITY **Myth:** Standing on your head or thrusting up your hips for half an hour after sex will help you get pregnant. **Reality:** If you're having sex at your fertile time of the month, the sperm will arrive at their destination no matter your position.

Friday ___ / ___

CYCLE DAY ☐   PRENATAL SUPPLEMENT ☐

OVULATION / PREGNANCY SIGNS

TESTS / MEDS / PROCEDURES
_____
_____
_____
_____

EXERCISE
_____
_____
_____

RELAXATION
_____
_____
_____

NOTES

Saturday ___ / ___

CYCLE DAY ☐   PRENATAL SUPPLEMENT ☐

OVULATION / PREGNANCY SIGNS

TESTS / MEDS / PROCEDURES
_____
_____
_____
_____

EXERCISE
_____
_____
_____

RELAXATION
_____
_____
_____

NOTES

THROUGH THE AGES The first successful artificial insemination via donor sperm occurred in 1884—*without* the woman's knowledge. While ostensibly performing a routine exam, a doctor inseminated his patient with a handsome med student's sperm. He never saw fit to tell the woman, but did eventually inform her infertile husband.

Sunday ___/___

CYCLE DAY ☐   PRENATAL SUPPLEMENT ☐

OVULATION / PREGNANCY SIGNS

TESTS / MEDS / PROCEDURES

_____
_____
_____
_____
_____

EXERCISE

_____
_____
_____
_____

RELAXATION

_____
_____
_____
_____

NOTES

Week in Review

GOAL CHECK _____

TOTAL EXERCISE SESSIONS _____

TOTAL RELAXATION SESSIONS_____

THOUGHTS AND FEELINGS

WEEK
5

DATES: _____

GOALS: _____
_____
_____
_____

Monday   __/__

CYCLE DAY [ ]   PRENATAL SUPPLEMENT [ ]

OVULATION / PREGNANCY SIGNS

TESTS / MEDS / PROCEDURES
_____
_____
_____
_____
_____

EXERCISE
_____
_____
_____

RELAXATION
_____
_____
_____

NOTES

Tuesday   __/__

CYCLE DAY [ ]   PRENATAL SUPPLEMENT [ ]

OVULATION / PREGNANCY SIGNS

TESTS / MEDS / PROCEDURES
_____
_____
_____
_____
_____

EXERCISE
_____
_____
_____

RELAXATION
_____
_____
_____

NOTES

BY THE NUMBERS   **200 million:** Approximate number of sperm deposited into the vagina near the cervix in a typical ejaculation. **100,000:** Number of sperm that make it into the uterus—less than 0.1 percent. **400:** The number of sperm that reach the immediate vicinity of the egg.

Wednesday   __/__

CYCLE DAY ☐   PRENATAL SUPPLEMENT ☐

OVULATION / PREGNANCY SIGNS

TESTS / MEDS / PROCEDURES

EXERCISE

RELAXATION

NOTES

Thursday   __/__

CYCLE DAY ☐   PRENATAL SUPPLEMENT ☐

OVULATION / PREGNANCY SIGNS

TESTS / MEDS / PROCEDURES

EXERCISE

RELAXATION

NOTES

CONCEPTION WONDERS   In 2004, a healthy British baby was born using sperm that had been frozen for 21 years, apparently a world record. Thawed animal sperm has been used successfully for up to 40 years after it was frozen.

Friday

__/__

CYCLE DAY ☐   PRENATAL SUPPLEMENT ☐

OVULATION / PREGNANCY SIGNS

TESTS / MEDS / PROCEDURES

EXERCISE

RELAXATION

NOTES

Saturday

__/__

CYCLE DAY ☐   PRENATAL SUPPLEMENT ☐

OVULATION / PREGNANCY SIGNS

TESTS / MEDS / PROCEDURES

EXERCISE

RELAXATION

NOTES

THROUGH THE AGES   A 1969 Harris poll found more than half of Americans believed that emerging reproductive technologies such as artificial insemination, in-vitro fertilization, and surrogate motherhood would "encourage promiscuity" and signify "the end of babies born through love."

Sunday   __/__   CYCLE ☐   PRENATAL ☐
                                       DAY   SUPPLEMENT

OVULATION / PREGNANCY SIGNS

TESTS / MEDS / PROCEDURES

_____

_____

_____

_____

_____

EXERCISE

_____

_____

_____

RELAXATION

_____

_____

_____

NOTES

Week in Review

GOAL CHECK _____

TOTAL EXERCISE SESSIONS _____

TOTAL RELAXATION SESSIONS _____

THOUGHTS AND FEELINGS

WEEK
6

DATES: _____

GOALS: _____

_____

_____

_____

Monday   __/__

CYCLE DAY [ ]   PRENATAL SUPPLEMENT [ ]

OVULATION / PREGNANCY SIGNS

TESTS / MEDS / PROCEDURES

_____

_____

_____

_____

_____

EXERCISE

_____

_____

_____

NOTES

RELAXATION

_____

_____

_____

Tuesday   __/__

CYCLE DAY [ ]   PRENATAL SUPPLEMENT [ ]

OVULATION / PREGNANCY SIGNS

TESTS / MEDS / PROCEDURES

_____

_____

_____

_____

EXERCISE

_____

_____

_____

NOTES

RELAXATION

_____

_____

_____

BY THE NUMBERS **2.6:** Average number of children per Utah woman, the highest U.S. average. **1.7:** Average births per female residents of Maine, Massachusetts, and Vermont. **7.5:** Average number of children per women in Niger, Africa, home of the world's highest fertility rate. **1.3:** Birth rates in Spain and Italy.

Wednesday   __/__

CYCLE DAY [ ]   PRENATAL SUPPLEMENT [ ]

OVULATION / PREGNANCY SIGNS

TESTS / MEDS / PROCEDURES

EXERCISE

NOTES

RELAXATION

Thursday   __/__

CYCLE DAY [ ]   PRENATAL SUPPLEMENT [ ]

OVULATION / PREGNANCY SIGNS

TESTS / MEDS / PROCEDURES

EXERCISE

NOTES

RELAXATION

MYTH VS. REALITY **Myth:** Boxer shorts are better for a man's sperm count than briefs. **Reality:** Whether a man wears boxers or briefs, his scrotal temperature will average from 94° to 95°F, the ideal temperature for healthy sperm production. Still, men seeking to preserve their fertility should limit time spent in saunas and hot tubs.

Friday ___/___

CYCLE DAY ☐   PRENATAL SUPPLEMENT ☐

OVULATION / PREGNANCY SIGNS

TESTS / MEDS / PROCEDURES
_____
_____
_____
_____
_____

EXERCISE
_____
_____
_____

NOTES

RELAXATION
_____
_____
_____

Saturday ___/___

CYCLE DAY ☐   PRENATAL SUPPLEMENT ☐

OVULATION / PREGNANCY SIGNS

TESTS / MEDS / PROCEDURES
_____
_____
_____
_____
_____

EXERCISE
_____
_____
_____

NOTES

RELAXATION
_____
_____
_____

THROUGH THE AGES   Some nineteenth-century physicians believed that infertility was caused by a woman's "excessive or luxurious living" or by strenuous mental activity such as schooling. "The results are monstrous brains and puny bodies," a Harvard physician wrote. "The brain cannot take more than its share without injury to other organs."

Sunday   __/__   CYCLE DAY ☐   PRENATAL SUPPLEMENT ☐

OVULATION / PREGNANCY SIGNS

TESTS / MEDS / PROCEDURES

_____
_____
_____
_____
_____

EXERCISE

_____
_____
_____

RELAXATION

_____
_____
_____

NOTES

Week in Review

GOAL CHECK _____

TOTAL EXERCISE SESSIONS _____

TOTAL RELAXATION SESSIONS _____

THOUGHTS AND FEELINGS

WEEK
7

DATES: _____

GOALS: _____

_____

_____

_____

Monday   __/__

CYCLE DAY [ ]   PRENATAL SUPPLEMENT [ ]

OVULATION / PREGNANCY SIGNS

TESTS / MEDS / PROCEDURES

_____

_____

_____

_____

EXERCISE

_____

_____

_____

_____

RELAXATION

_____

_____

_____

_____

NOTES

Tuesday   __/__

CYCLE DAY [ ]   PRENATAL SUPPLEMENT [ ]

OVULATION / PREGNANCY SIGNS

TESTS / MEDS / PROCEDURES

_____

_____

_____

_____

EXERCISE

_____

_____

_____

_____

RELAXATION

_____

_____

_____

_____

NOTES

BY THE NUMBERS **2:** Number of cells an embryo has within 38 hours of penetration by the sperm. **8:** Typical number of cells that an embryo has after 3 days of development. **64 to 160:** Number of cells an embryo has by Day 5, when it passes from the fallopian tubes into the uterus.

Wednesday __/__

CYCLE DAY ☐   PRENATAL SUPPLEMENT ☐

OVULATION / PREGNANCY SIGNS

TESTS / MEDS / PROCEDURES

EXERCISE

NOTES

RELAXATION

Thursday __/__

CYCLE DAY ☐   PRENATAL SUPPLEMENT ☐

OVULATION / PREGNANCY SIGNS

TESTS / MEDS / PROCEDURES

EXERCISE

NOTES

RELAXATION

CONCEPTION WONDERS DNA testing in paternity cases has proven numerous cases of fraternal twins fathered by different men. So-called "heteropaternal super-fecundation" happens when a woman produces two eggs that are fertilized by sperm from different sexual partners, typically within 24 hours.

Friday __/__

CYCLE DAY ☐   PRENATAL SUPPLEMENT ☐

OVULATION / PREGNANCY SIGNS

TESTS / MEDS / PROCEDURES

EXERCISE

RELAXATION

NOTES

Saturday __/__

CYCLE DAY ☐   PRENATAL SUPPLEMENT ☐

OVULATION / PREGNANCY SIGNS

TESTS / MEDS / PROCEDURES

EXERCISE

RELAXATION

NOTES

THROUGH THE AGES The phrase "the rabbit died" became a euphemism for a positive pregnancy test in the late 1920s, when it was discovered that injecting a pregnant woman's urine into a rabbit would produce bulging masses on the rabbit's ovaries. These masses couldn't be seen without killing the rabbit.

Sunday   __/__

CYCLE DAY ☐   PRENATAL SUPPLEMENT ☐

OVULATION / PREGNANCY SIGNS

TESTS / MEDS / PROCEDURES

_____
_____
_____
_____
_____

EXERCISE

_____
_____
_____
_____

NOTES

RELAXATION

_____
_____
_____
_____

Week in Review

GOAL CHECK _____
TOTAL EXERCISE SESSIONS _____
TOTAL RELAXATION SESSIONS_____

THOUGHTS AND FEELINGS

WEEK
8

DATES: _____

GOALS: _____

_____

_____

_____

Monday   __/__

CYCLE DAY ☐   PRENATAL SUPPLEMENT ☐

OVULATION / PREGNANCY SIGNS

TESTS / MEDS / PROCEDURES

_____

_____

_____

_____

_____

EXERCISE

_____

_____

_____

_____

RELAXATION

_____

_____

_____

_____

NOTES

Tuesday   __/__

CYCLE DAY ☐   PRENATAL SUPPLEMENT ☐

OVULATION / PREGNANCY SIGNS

TESTS / MEDS / PROCEDURES

_____

_____

_____

_____

_____

EXERCISE

_____

_____

_____

_____

RELAXATION

_____

_____

_____

_____

NOTES

BY THE NUMBERS **74:** Percent increase in twin births from 1980 to 2000, due to increases in fertility treatments and the delayed age of birth mothers. Older women are more likely to have multiples than younger women. **3:** Percent of all babies who were born as a twin or higher-order multiples in 2000. **1.2:** Historical rate of twin pregnancies.

Wednesday ___/___

CYCLE DAY ☐   PRENATAL SUPPLEMENT ☐

OVULATION / PREGNANCY SIGNS

TESTS / MEDS / PROCEDURES

EXERCISE

NOTES

RELAXATION

Thursday ___/___

CYCLE DAY ☐   PRENATAL SUPPLEMENT ☐

OVULATION / PREGNANCY SIGNS

TESTS / MEDS / PROCEDURES

EXERCISE

NOTES

RELAXATION

MYTH VS. REALITY   **Myth:** A couple's conception difficulties usually can be traced to the woman. **Reality:** Only about half of fertility problems are due to female-factor problems, and 40 percent are due to male fertility problems. About 10 percent are unexplained. Yet even as late as the nineteenth century, some physicians still refused to consider the possibility that male factors played a role in infertility at all.

Friday   __/__

CYCLE DAY ☐   PRENATAL SUPPLEMENT ☐

OVULATION / PREGNANCY SIGNS

TESTS / MEDS / PROCEDURES

EXERCISE

NOTES

RELAXATION

Saturday   __/__

CYCLE DAY ☐   PRENATAL SUPPLEMENT ☐

OVULATION / PREGNANCY SIGNS

TESTS / MEDS / PROCEDURES

EXERCISE

NOTES

RELAXATION

THROUGH THE AGES   In medieval Europe, tradition held that a man who dreamed of having a son would place a battle-axe under a pillow; at climax, he'd retrieve it and exclaim to his wife: "You must have a boy." If he wanted a daughter, he'd place a hat on his wife's head and whisper tender words to her.

Sunday ___/___

CYCLE DAY ☐   PRENATAL SUPPLEMENT ☐

OVULATION / PREGNANCY SIGNS

TESTS / MEDS / PROCEDURES

_____
_____
_____
_____
_____

EXERCISE

_____
_____
_____
_____

RELAXATION

_____
_____
_____
_____

NOTES

Week in Review

GOAL CHECK _____

TOTAL EXERCISE SESSIONS _____

TOTAL RELAXATION SESSIONS _____

THOUGHTS AND FEELINGS

WEEK
9

DATES: _____

GOALS: _____

_____

_____

_____

Monday   __/__

CYCLE DAY [ ]   PRENATAL SUPPLEMENT [ ]

OVULATION / PREGNANCY SIGNS

TESTS / MEDS / PROCEDURES

_____

_____

_____

_____

_____

EXERCISE

_____

_____

_____

RELAXATION

_____

_____

_____

NOTES

Tuesday   __/__

CYCLE DAY [ ]   PRENATAL SUPPLEMENT [ ]

OVULATION / PREGNANCY SIGNS

TESTS / MEDS / PROCEDURES

_____

_____

_____

_____

_____

EXERCISE

_____

_____

_____

RELAXATION

_____

_____

_____

NOTES

BY THE NUMBERS   **–196°C:** Temperature at which frozen sperm are stored. **2:** Number of hours it takes to freeze sperm, cooling them at 0.3 to 2 degrees per minute. **15:** Number of minutes required to thaw sperm.

Wednesday   __/__

CYCLE DAY ☐   PRENATAL SUPPLEMENT ☐

OVULATION / PREGNANCY SIGNS

TESTS / MEDS / PROCEDURES

EXERCISE

RELAXATION

NOTES

Thursday   __/__

CYCLE DAY ☐   PRENATAL SUPPLEMENT ☐

OVULATION / PREGNANCY SIGNS

TESTS / MEDS / PROCEDURES

EXERCISE

RELAXATION

NOTES

CONCEPTION WONDERS   In 2005, a 66-year-old Romanian woman gave birth to a girl conceived using donor eggs and donor sperm, becoming the world's oldest birth mom. In 2006, a 59-year-old New York woman became the world's oldest woman to deliver twins, via donor eggs and her husband's sperm.

Friday   —/—

CYCLE DAY ☐   PRENATAL SUPPLEMENT ☐

OVULATION / PREGNANCY SIGNS

TESTS / MEDS / PROCEDURES

EXERCISE

RELAXATION

NOTES

Saturday   —/—

CYCLE DAY ☐   PRENATAL SUPPLEMENT ☐

OVULATION / PREGNANCY SIGNS

TESTS / MEDS / PROCEDURES

EXERCISE

NOTES

RELAXATION

THROUGH THE AGES In a 1909 medical journal article about artificial insemination, a doctor maintained that children are formed entirely by the mother's genetic contribution. He considered it a "scientific fact" that the sperm donor "is of no more importance than the personality of the finger which pulls the trigger of a gun."

Sunday ___/___

CYCLE DAY ☐   PRENATAL SUPPLEMENT ☐

OVULATION / PREGNANCY SIGNS

TESTS / MEDS / PROCEDURES

_____
_____
_____
_____
_____

EXERCISE

_____
_____
_____
_____

RELAXATION

_____
_____
_____
_____

NOTES

Week in Review

GOAL CHECK _____
TOTAL EXERCISE SESSIONS _____
TOTAL RELAXATION SESSIONS _____

THOUGHTS AND FEELINGS

WEEK
10

DATES: _____

GOALS: _____

_____

_____

_____

Monday ___/___

CYCLE DAY [ ]   PRENATAL SUPPLEMENT [ ]

OVULATION / PREGNANCY SIGNS

TESTS / MEDS / PROCEDURES

_____

_____

_____

_____

_____

EXERCISE

_____

_____

_____

RELAXATION

_____

_____

_____

_____

NOTES

Tuesday ___/___

CYCLE DAY [ ]   PRENATAL SUPPLEMENT [ ]

OVULATION / PREGNANCY SIGNS

TESTS / MEDS / PROCEDURES

_____

_____

_____

_____

_____

EXERCISE

_____

_____

_____

RELAXATION

_____

_____

_____

NOTES

BY THE NUMBERS **100 million:** Average number of sperm in a fertile man's ejaculate. **10 billion:** Average number of sperm in a bull's ejaculate, though the volume of the bull's ejaculate is no greater than that of a man. Bull sperm move at three times the speed of the human sperm, and virtually none are abnormal or weak.

Wednesday ___/___

CYCLE DAY ☐   PRENATAL SUPPLEMENT ☐

OVULATION / PREGNANCY SIGNS

TESTS / MEDS / PROCEDURES

EXERCISE

RELAXATION

NOTES

Thursday ___/___

CYCLE DAY ☐   PRENATAL SUPPLEMENT ☐

OVULATION / PREGNANCY SIGNS

TESTS / MEDS / PROCEDURES

EXERCISE

RELAXATION

NOTES

MYTH VS. REALITY **Myth:** The propensity for having identical twins is primarily genetic. **Reality:** The chance of having identical twins is mostly just chance, though there may be some slight genetic mechanism. The odds of having fraternal twins, unassisted by fertility drugs, are linked to a genetic predisposition to release multiple eggs.

Friday ___/___

CYCLE DAY ☐   PRENATAL SUPPLEMENT ☐

OVULATION / PREGNANCY SIGNS

TESTS / MEDS / PROCEDURES

_____
_____
_____
_____
_____

EXERCISE

_____
_____
_____

RELAXATION

_____
_____
_____
_____

NOTES

Saturday ___/___

CYCLE DAY ☐   PRENATAL SUPPLEMENT ☐

OVULATION / PREGNANCY SIGNS

TESTS / MEDS / PROCEDURES

_____
_____
_____
_____
_____

EXERCISE

_____
_____
_____

RELAXATION

_____
_____
_____

NOTES

THROUGH THE AGES   In 1992, Cecil Jacobson, a Virginia physician and fertility specialist known as "The Sperminator," was convicted on 53 counts of fraud and perjury and sentenced to five years in prison. Instead of finding sperm donors for his patients, he used his own sperm, fathering as many as 75 children.

Sunday __/__

CYCLE DAY ☐   PRENATAL SUPPLEMENT ☐

OVULATION / PREGNANCY SIGNS

TESTS / MEDS / PROCEDURES

_____
_____
_____
_____
_____

EXERCISE

_____
_____
_____
_____

RELAXATION

_____
_____
_____
_____

NOTES

Week in Review

GOAL CHECK _____

TOTAL EXERCISE SESSIONS _____

TOTAL RELAXATION SESSIONS _____

THOUGHTS AND FEELINGS

WEEK
11

DATES: _____

GOALS: _____

_____

_____

_____

Monday

__/__

CYCLE DAY ☐

PRENATAL SUPPLEMENT ☐

OVULATION / PREGNANCY SIGNS

TESTS / MEDS / PROCEDURES

_____

_____

_____

_____

_____

EXERCISE

_____

_____

_____

RELAXATION

_____

_____

_____

NOTES

Tuesday

__/__

CYCLE DAY ☐

PRENATAL SUPPLEMENT ☐

OVULATION / PREGNANCY SIGNS

TESTS / MEDS / PROCEDURES

_____

_____

_____

_____

_____

EXERCISE

_____

_____

_____

RELAXATION

_____

_____

_____

NOTES

BY THE NUMBERS **32:** Percent of IVF pregnancies that produce twins. **8 to 10:** Percent of Clomid pregnancies that produce twins. **1.7:** Percent of natural pregnancies that produce fraternal twins. **0.4:** Percent of pregnancies that produce identical twins.

Wednesday __/__

CYCLE DAY ☐   PRENATAL SUPPLEMENT ☐

OVULATION / PREGNANCY SIGNS

TESTS / MEDS / PROCEDURES

EXERCISE

RELAXATION

NOTES

Thursday __/__

CYCLE DAY ☐   PRENATAL SUPPLEMENT ☐

OVULATION / PREGNANCY SIGNS

TESTS / MEDS / PROCEDURES

EXERCISE

RELAXATION

NOTES

CONCEPTION WONDERS   A North Carolina man was 94 years old when he fathered a child with his 27-year-old wife, according to a 1935 article in the *Journal of the American Medical Association*. The article's authors pronounced the man's sperm motility "very great," but they did not attempt to verify that this "hale and hearty figure" was indeed the father of his wife's baby.

Friday   __/__   CYCLE DAY ☐   PRENATAL SUPPLEMENT ☐

OVULATION / PREGNANCY SIGNS

TESTS / MEDS / PROCEDURES

EXERCISE

RELAXATION

NOTES

Saturday   __/__   CYCLE DAY ☐   PRENATAL SUPPLEMENT ☐

OVULATION / PREGNANCY SIGNS

TESTS / MEDS / PROCEDURES

EXERCISE

RELAXATION

NOTES

THROUGH THE AGES   The United States was the third country, after England and Australia, to produce a baby through in-vitro fertilization. Elizabeth Jordan Carr, the country's first "test tube" baby, born in 1981 in Norfolk, Virginia, was the world's fifteenth IVF baby.

Sunday

__/__

CYCLE DAY ☐   PRENATAL SUPPLEMENT ☐

OVULATION / PREGNANCY SIGNS

TESTS / MEDS / PROCEDURES

_____
_____
_____
_____
_____

EXERCISE

_____
_____
_____
_____

RELAXATION

_____
_____
_____

NOTES

Week in Review

GOAL CHECK _____

TOTAL EXERCISE SESSIONS _____

TOTAL RELAXATION SESSIONS _____

THOUGHTS AND FEELINGS

WEEK
12

DATES: _____

GOALS: _____

_____

_____

_____

Monday   __/__

CYCLE DAY [ ]   PRENATAL SUPPLEMENT [ ]

OVULATION / PREGNANCY SIGNS

TESTS / MEDS / PROCEDURES

_____

_____

_____

_____

_____

EXERCISE

_____

_____

_____

RELAXATION

_____

_____

_____

_____

NOTES

Tuesday   __/__

CYCLE DAY [ ]   PRENATAL SUPPLEMENT [ ]

OVULATION / PREGNANCY SIGNS

TESTS / MEDS / PROCEDURES

_____

_____

_____

_____

EXERCISE

_____

_____

_____

RELAXATION

_____

_____

_____

NOTES

BY THE NUMBERS **97:** Percent chance of conception within one year for women in their early twenties. **86:** Percent chance within a year for women in their late twenties. **72:** Percent chance for women in their early thirties. **65:** Percent chance for women in their late thirties.

Wednesday __/__

CYCLE DAY ☐   PRENATAL SUPPLEMENT ☐

OVULATION / PREGNANCY SIGNS

TESTS / MEDS / PROCEDURES

_____
_____
_____
_____
_____

EXERCICE

_____
_____
_____
_____

RELAXATION

_____
_____
_____
_____

NOTES

Thursday __/__

CYCLE DAY ☐   PRENATAL SUPPLEMENT ☐

OVULATION / PREGNANCY SIGNS

TESTS / MEDS / PROCEDURES

_____
_____
_____
_____
_____

EXERCISE

_____
_____
_____
_____

RELAXATION

_____
_____
_____
_____

NOTES

MYTH VS. REALITY **Myth:** Taking your morning temperature is a good way to time sex for conception. **Reality:** By the time your temperature spikes, ovulation has already occurred, and it's too late to conceive. An ovulation predictor kit alerts you *before* ovulation occurs.

Friday
—/—

CYCLE DAY ☐   PRENATAL SUPPLEMENT ☐

OVULATION / PREGNANCY SIGNS

TESTS / MEDS / PROCEDURES

EXERCISE

RELAXATION

NOTES

Saturday
—/—

CYCLE DAY ☐   PRENATAL SUPPLEMENT ☐

OVULATION / PREGNANCY SIGNS

TESTS / MEDS / PROCEDURES

EXERCISE

RELAXATION

NOTES

THROUGH THE AGES Not one child was born for an entire decade in a small Chinese village beginning in the mid-1920s. Later it was discovered that the cause of the "curse" was a switch in cooking oil, from soybean oil to a cheaper, crude cottonseed oil. A chemical in un-preheated cottonseed oil dramatically halts sperm production.

Sunday ___/___

CYCLE DAY ☐   PRENATAL SUPPLEMENT ☐

OVULATION / PREGNANCY SIGNS

TESTS / MEDS / PROCEDURES

_____
_____
_____
_____
_____

EXERCISE

_____
_____
_____

RELAXATION

_____
_____
_____
_____

NOTES

Week in Review

GOAL CHECK _____

TOTAL EXERCISE SESSIONS _____

TOTAL RELAXATION SESSIONS _____

THOUGHTS AND FEELINGS

WEEK
13

DATES: _____

GOALS: _____
_____
_____
_____
_____

Monday

___/___

CYCLE DAY [ ]   PRENATAL SUPPLEMENT [ ]

OVULATION / PREGNANCY SIGNS

TESTS / MEDS / PROCEDURES
_____
_____
_____
_____
_____

EXERCISE
_____
_____
_____

RELAXATION
_____
_____
_____
_____

NOTES

Tuesday

___/___

CYCLE DAY [ ]   PRENATAL SUPPLEMENT [ ]

OVULATION / PREGNANCY SIGNS

TESTS / MEDS / PROCEDURES
_____
_____
_____
_____
_____

EXERCISE
_____
_____
_____

RELAXATION
_____
_____
_____

NOTES

BY THE NUMBERS **72:** Approximate number of days it takes to complete production of a single sperm. **1 million:** Number of sperm that can be produced by a man each day. **40:** Typical percentage of abnormally shaped sperm in a normal human semen specimen.

Wednesday ___/___

CYCLE DAY ☐   PRENATAL SUPPLEMENT ☐

OVULATION / PREGNANCY SIGNS

TESTS / MEDS / PROCEDURES

EXERCISE

RELAXATION

NOTES

Thursday ___/___

CYCLE DAY ☐   PRENATAL SUPPLEMENT ☐

OVULATION / PREGNANCY SIGNS

TESTS / MEDS / PROCEDURES

EXERCISE

RELAXATION

NOTES

CONCEPTION WONDERS In 2004, Belgian doctors reported the first birth from frozen ovarian tissue. A cancer survivor, who'd had pieces of her ovaries surgically removed and frozen seven years earlier, gave birth after doctors transplanted the ovarian tissue back into her abdomen.

Friday   __/__

CYCLE DAY ☐   PRENATAL SUPPLEMENT ☐

OVULATION / PREGNANCY SIGNS

TESTS / MEDS / PROCEDURES

EXERCISE

RELAXATION

NOTES

Saturday   __/__

CYCLE DAY ☐   PRENATAL SUPPLEMENT ☐

OVULATION / PREGNANCY SIGNS

TESTS / MEDS / PROCEDURES

EXERCISE

RELAXATION

NOTES

THROUGH THE AGES In 1976, a New York con man announced plans to auction sperm from a "celebrity sperm bank"; donors supposedly included Mick Jagger, Bob Dylan, and John Lennon. Later, the prankster claimed the sperm had been stolen. Television shows reported the cancelled auction without realizing it had been a hoax.

Sunday
___/___

CYCLE DAY ☐   PRENATAL SUPPLEMENT ☐

OVULATION / PREGNANCY SIGNS

TESTS / MEDS / PROCEDURES

EXERCISE

RELAXATION

NOTES

Week in Review

GOAL CHECK _____

TOTAL EXERCISE SESSIONS _____

TOTAL RELAXATION SESSIONS_____

THOUGHTS AND FEELINGS

WEEK
14

DATES: _____

GOALS: _____

_____

_____

_____

Monday

__/__

CYCLE DAY [ ] PRENATAL SUPPLEMENT [ ]

OVULATION / PREGNANCY SIGNS

TESTS / MEDS / PROCEDURES

_____

_____

_____

_____

_____

EXERCISE

_____

_____

_____

RELAXATION

_____

_____

_____

NOTES

Tuesday

__/__

CYCLE DAY [ ] PRENATAL SUPPLEMENT [ ]

OVULATION / PREGNANCY SIGNS

TESTS / MEDS / PROCEDURES

_____

_____

_____

_____

_____

EXERCISE

_____

_____

_____

RELAXATION

_____

_____

_____

NOTES

BY THE NUMBERS **4:** The average number of births per woman in the United States in 1900. **2.2:** The fertility rate during the Great Depression. **3.7:** The postwar fertility rate, peaking in 1957. **2.0:** Average births per U.S. woman over the last 20 years.

Wednesday ___/___

CYCLE DAY ☐   PRENATAL SUPPLEMENT ☐

OVULATION / PREGNANCY SIGNS

TESTS / MEDS / PROCEDURES

_____
_____
_____
_____
_____

EXERCISE

_____
_____
_____

NOTES

RELAXATION

_____
_____
_____
_____

Thursday ___/___

CYCLE DAY ☐   PRENATAL SUPPLEMENT ☐

OVULATION / PREGNANCY SIGNS

TESTS / MEDS / PROCEDURES

_____
_____
_____
_____
_____

EXERCISE

_____
_____
_____

NOTES

RELAXATION

_____
_____
_____
_____

MYTH VS. REALITY **Myth:** The human sperm count is declining. **Reality:** Average American sperm counts today are not significantly different from 50 years ago. However, the human sperm count has been declining over hundreds of thousands of years, an evolutionary trend related to our monogamous mating pattern.

Friday   __/__

CYCLE DAY [ ]   PRENATAL SUPPLEMENT [ ]

OVULATION / PREGNANCY SIGNS

TESTS / MEDS / PROCEDURES

_____
_____
_____
_____
_____

EXERCISE

_____
_____
_____

NOTES

RELAXATION

_____
_____
_____

Saturday   __/__

CYCLE DAY [ ]   PRENATAL SUPPLEMENT [ ]

OVULATION / PREGNANCY SIGNS

TESTS / MEDS / PROCEDURES

_____
_____
_____
_____
_____

EXERCISE

_____
_____
_____

NOTES

RELAXATION

_____
_____
_____

THROUGH THE AGES In 1948, a British commission recommended that artificial insemination using donor sperm (AID) be made a criminal offense. "Succession through blood descent," the commission wrote, "is at the basis of our society. On it depend . . . titles of honour, and the Monarchy itself." The British Medical Association considered AID "an offense against society."

Sunday ___/___

CYCLE DAY ☐ PRENATAL SUPPLEMENT ☐

OVULATION / PREGNANCY SIGNS

TESTS / MEDS / PROCEDURES
_____
_____
_____
_____
_____

EXERCISE
_____
_____
_____
_____

RELAXATION
_____
_____
_____
_____

NOTES

Week in Review

GOAL CHECK _____

TOTAL EXERCISE SESSIONS _____

TOTAL RELAXATION SESSIONS _____

THOUGHTS AND FEELINGS

WEEK
15

DATES: _____

GOALS: _____

_____

_____

_____

Monday

___/___

CYCLE DAY ☐

PRENATAL SUPPLEMENT ☐

OVULATION / PREGNANCY SIGNS

TESTS / MEDS / PROCEDURES

_____

_____

_____

_____

_____

EXERCISE

_____

_____

_____

RELAXATION

_____

_____

_____

_____

NOTES

Tuesday

___/___

CYCLE DAY ☐

PRENATAL SUPPLEMENT ☐

OVULATION / PREGNANCY SIGNS

TESTS / MEDS / PROCEDURES

_____

_____

_____

_____

_____

EXERCISE

_____

_____

_____

RELAXATION

_____

_____

_____

_____

NOTES

BY THE NUMBERS   **48:** Percent of nonsmokers who got pregnant via IVF in a Canadian study. **20:** Percent of nonsmokers who lived with smokers and got pregnant. **19:** Percent of smokers who got pregnant. Research suggests that smoking adds 10 years to a woman's reproductive "age" and increases miscarriage rate.

Wednesday   __/__

CYCLE DAY ☐   PRENATAL SUPPLEMENT ☐

OVULATION / PREGNANCY SIGNS

TESTS / MEDS / PROCEDURES

EXERCISE

NOTES

RELAXATION

Thursday   __/__

CYCLE DAY ☐   PRENATAL SUPPLEMENT ☐

OVULATION / PREGNANCY SIGNS

TESTS / MEDS / PROCEDURES

EXERCISE

NOTES

RELAXATION

CONCEPTION WONDERS In 1999 and 2000, a mother in New Zealand, Jayne Bleackley, gave birth to children just 208 days apart, setting the record for the shortest interval between two children born in separate pregnancies.

Friday

___/___

CYCLE DAY ☐   PRENATAL SUPPLEMENT ☐

OVULATION / PREGNANCY SIGNS

TESTS / MEDS / PROCEDURES

_____
_____
_____
_____
_____

EXERCISE

_____
_____
_____

RELAXATION

_____
_____
_____

NOTES

Saturday

___/___

CYCLE DAY ☐   PRENATAL SUPPLEMENT ☐

OVULATION / PREGNANCY SIGNS

TESTS / MEDS / PROCEDURES

_____
_____
_____
_____

EXERCISE

_____
_____
_____

RELAXATION

_____
_____

NOTES

THROUGH THE AGES In a fertility treatment practiced by ancient Egyptians, a woman would squat over a hot mixture of frankincense, oil, dates, and beer and allow the vapors to enter her. One pregnancy test involved mixing melon puree with the milk of a woman who'd delivered a boy. If the concoction made the woman sick, she was thought to be pregnant.

Sunday   __/__   CYCLE ☐   PRENATAL ☐
                                           DAY   SUPPLEMENT

OVULATION / PREGNANCY SIGNS   TESTS / MEDS / PROCEDURES

EXERCISE

NOTES

RELAXATION

Week in Review

GOAL CHECK _____

TOTAL EXERCISE SESSIONS _____

TOTAL RELAXATION SESSIONS_____

THOUGHTS AND FEELINGS

WEEK

16

DATES: _____

GOALS: _____
_____
_____
_____

Monday
___/___

CYCLE DAY ☐   PRENATAL SUPPLEMENT ☐

OVULATION / PREGNANCY SIGNS

TESTS / MEDS / PROCEDURES
_____
_____
_____
_____
_____

EXERCISE
_____
_____
_____

NOTES

RELAXATION
_____
_____
_____
_____

Tuesday
___/___

CYCLE DAY ☐   PRENATAL SUPPLEMENT ☐

OVULATION / PREGNANCY SIGNS

TESTS / MEDS / PROCEDURES
_____
_____
_____
_____
_____

EXERCISE
_____
_____
_____

NOTES

RELAXATION
_____
_____
_____
_____

BY THE NUMBERS **1/5:** The rate at which vegan women give birth to fraternal twins compared to women who do eat animal products, particularly dairy. This may be because vegan women have lower blood levels of a protein, found in milk, that makes the ovaries more sensitive to follicle stimulating hormones.

Wednesday ___/___

CYCLE DAY ☐   PRENATAL SUPPLEMENT ☐

OVULATION / PREGNANCY SIGNS

TESTS / MEDS / PROCEDURES

_____
_____
_____
_____
_____

EXERCISE

_____
_____
_____
_____

RELAXATION

_____
_____
_____
_____

NOTES

Thursday ___/___

CYCLE DAY ☐   PRENATAL SUPPLEMENT ☐

OVULATION / PREGNANCY SIGNS

TESTS / MEDS / PROCEDURES

_____
_____
_____
_____
_____

EXERCISE

_____
_____
_____
_____

RELAXATION

_____
_____
_____
_____

NOTES

MYTH VS. REALITY **Myth:** A normal menstrual cycle is 28 days. **Reality:** "Normal" cycles can range from about 24 days to 36 days and vary from woman to woman as well as within individuals. You can ovulate as early as Day 8 and as late as Day 22 or beyond.

Friday

___/___

| CYCLE DAY | | PRENATAL SUPPLEMENT | |

OVULATION / PREGNANCY SIGNS

TESTS / MEDS / PROCEDURES

_____
_____
_____
_____
_____

EXERCISE

_____
_____
_____

RELAXATION

_____
_____
_____

NOTES

Saturday

___/___

| CYCLE DAY | | PRENATAL SUPPLEMENT | |

OVULATION / PREGNANCY SIGNS

TESTS / MEDS / PROCEDURES

_____
_____
_____
_____
_____

EXERCISE

_____
_____
_____

RELAXATION

_____
_____
_____

NOTES

THROUGH THE AGES Sperm were discovered in 1677, when a Dutchman used a microscope to examine the nocturnal emissions of an ill man and declared the fluid was "alive." A colleague then examined his own semen, proposing that sperm were the source of reproduction, not evidence of disease.

Sunday ___/___

CYCLE DAY ☐   PRENATAL SUPPLEMENT ☐

OVULATION / PREGNANCY SIGNS

TESTS / MEDS / PROCEDURES

EXERCISE

RELAXATION

NOTES

Week in Review

GOAL CHECK _____

TOTAL EXERCISE SESSIONS _____

TOTAL RELAXATION SESSIONS _____

THOUGHTS AND FEELINGS

WEEK
17

DATES: _____

GOALS: _____
_____
_____
_____
_____

Monday   __/__

CYCLE DAY ☐   PRENATAL SUPPLEMENT ☐

OVULATION / PREGNANCY SIGNS

TESTS / MEDS / PROCEDURES
_____
_____
_____
_____
_____

EXERCISE
_____
_____
_____
_____

NOTES

RELAXATION
_____
_____
_____
_____

Tuesday   __/__

CYCLE DAY ☐   PRENATAL SUPPLEMENT ☐

OVULATION / PREGNANCY SIGNS

TESTS / MEDS / PROCEDURES
_____
_____
_____
_____

EXERCISE
_____
_____
_____
_____

NOTES

RELAXATION
_____
_____
_____

BY THE NUMBERS   **3:** Percent of semen that is comprised of sperm. The rest is a media for the sperm to live in. **3 or 4:** The number of times a man actually ejaculates when he experiences an orgasm. The first contraction is the richest in sperm. **1 billion:** The number of sperm stored in the testicles.

Wednesday   __/__

CYCLE DAY ☐   PRENATAL SUPPLEMENT ☐

OVULATION / PREGNANCY SIGNS

TESTS / MEDS / PROCEDURES

_____
_____
_____
_____
_____

EXERCISE

_____
_____
_____
_____

NOTES

RELAXATION

_____
_____
_____
_____

Thursday   __/__

CYCLE DAY ☐   PRENATAL SUPPLEMENT ☐

OVULATION / PREGNANCY SIGNS

TESTS / MEDS / PROCEDURES

_____
_____
_____
_____
_____

EXERCISE

_____
_____
_____
_____

NOTES

RELAXATION

_____
_____
_____
_____

CONCEPTION WONDERS   A North Dakota woman gave birth to eight sets of fraternal twins beginning in the 1940s, and an Italian woman reportedly gave birth to 11 sets of twins, the last in 1947. The record for the most sets of twins—unconfirmed—is held by an eighteenth-century Russian woman who reportedly gave birth to 16 sets of twins.

Friday   —/—

CYCLE DAY ☐   PRENATAL SUPPLEMENT ☐

OVULATION / PREGNANCY SIGNS

TESTS / MEDS / PROCEDURES

_____
_____
_____
_____
_____

EXERCISE

_____
_____
_____

RELAXATION

_____
_____
_____

NOTES

Saturday   —/—

CYCLE DAY ☐   PRENATAL SUPPLEMENT ☐

OVULATION / PREGNANCY SIGNS

TESTS / MEDS / PROCEDURES

_____
_____
_____
_____

EXERCISE

_____
_____
_____

RELAXATION

_____

NOTES

THROUGH THE AGES The first home pregnancy test, marketed in 1978, took 2 hours and was 97 percent accurate for positive results, but only 80 percent accurate for negative results. The kit included a vial of purified water, a medicine dropper, and a test tube containing freeze-dried red blood cells from sheep.

Sunday   __/__

CYCLE DAY ☐   PRENATAL SUPPLEMENT ☐

OVULATION / PREGNANCY SIGNS

TESTS / MEDS / PROCEDURES

_____
_____
_____
_____
_____

EXERCISE

_____
_____
_____

RELAXATION

_____
_____
_____
_____

NOTES

Week in Review

GOAL CHECK _____

TOTAL EXERCISE SESSIONS _____

TOTAL RELAXATION SESSIONS_____

THOUGHTS AND FEELINGS

WEEK
18

DATES: _____

GOALS: _____

_____

_____

_____

Monday

__/__

CYCLE DAY ☐   PRENATAL SUPPLEMENT ☐

OVULATION / PREGNANCY SIGNS

TESTS / MEDS / PROCEDURES

EXERCISE

_____

_____

_____

RELAXATION

_____

_____

_____

NOTES

Tuesday

__/__

CYCLE DAY ☐   PRENATAL SUPPLEMENT ☐

OVULATION / PREGNANCY SIGNS

TESTS / MEDS / PROCEDURES

EXERCISE

_____

_____

_____

RELAXATION

_____

_____

_____

NOTES

BY THE NUMBERS **3:** Approximate number of hours required to freeze an embryo. **35:** Number of seconds it takes for frozen embryos to warm to room temperature. **40:** Number of minutes it takes to thaw a frozen embryo and prepare it for transfer.

Wednesday __/__

CYCLE DAY [ ]   PRENATAL SUPPLEMENT [ ]

OVULATION / PREGNANCY SIGNS

TESTS / MEDS / PROCEDURES

EXERCISE

NOTES

RELAXATION

Thursday __/__

CYCLE DAY [ ]   PRENATAL SUPPLEMENT [ ]

OVULATION / PREGNANCY SIGNS

TESTS / MEDS / PROCEDURES

EXERCISE

NOTES

RELAXATION

MYTH VS. REALITY   **Myth:** Your chances of getting pregnant are better if you have sex in the morning. **Reality:** Though some research suggests a man's sperm count may be higher in the morning, the differences are minimal, and there is no evidence showing that the differences affect conception odds.

Friday   __/__

CYCLE DAY [ ]   PRENATAL SUPPLEMENT [ ]

OVULATION / PREGNANCY SIGNS

TESTS / MEDS / PROCEDURES

_____
_____
_____
_____

EXERCISE

_____
_____
_____
_____

RELAXATION

_____
_____
_____
_____

NOTES

Saturday   __/__

CYCLE DAY [ ]   PRENATAL SUPPLEMENT [ ]

OVULATION / PREGNANCY SIGNS

TESTS / MEDS / PROCEDURES

_____
_____
_____
_____

EXERCISE

_____
_____
_____
_____

RELAXATION

_____
_____
_____
_____

NOTES

THROUGH THE AGES Though the first IVF baby was born in 1978 in England, the event might have happened four years earlier at a New York City hospital. However, when hospital officials learned of the IVF experiment, conducted on the sly by an eccentric fertility doctor, they destroyed the fertilized eggs.

Sunday ___/___

CYCLE DAY ☐   PRENATAL SUPPLEMENT ☐

OVULATION / PREGNANCY SIGNS

TESTS / MEDS / PROCEDURES
_____
_____
_____
_____
_____

EXERCISE
_____
_____
_____

RELAXATION
_____
_____
_____

NOTES

Week in Review

GOAL CHECK _____

TOTAL EXERCISE SESSIONS _____

TOTAL RELAXATION SESSIONS _____

THOUGHTS AND FEELINGS

WEEK

19

DATES: _____

GOALS: _____

_____

_____

_____

Monday

__/__

CYCLE DAY [ ]

PRENATAL SUPPLEMENT [ ]

OVULATION / PREGNANCY SIGNS

TESTS / MEDS / PROCEDURES

_____

_____

_____

_____

_____

EXERCISE

_____

_____

_____

NOTES

RELAXATION

_____

_____

_____

_____

Tuesday

__/__

CYCLE DAY [ ]

PRENATAL SUPPLEMENT [ ]

OVULATION / PREGNANCY SIGNS

TESTS / MEDS / PROCEDURES

_____

_____

_____

_____

_____

EXERCISE

_____

_____

_____

NOTES

RELAXATION

_____

_____

_____

_____

BY THE NUMBERS **1 in 22:** Odds of having fraternal twins among one tribe in Nigeria, the world's highest twin rate. **1 in 90:** Odds of having fraternal twins in the United States. **1 in 166:** Odds of having fraternal twins in Japan, the world's lowest rate. **1 in 12:** Odds of having a second set of fraternal twins if you already have one set.

Wednesday __/__

CYCLE DAY ☐   PRENATAL SUPPLEMENT ☐

OVULATION / PREGNANCY SIGNS

TESTS / MEDS / PROCEDURES

EXERCISE

RELAXATION

NOTES

Thursday __/__

CYCLE DAY ☐   PRENATAL SUPPLEMENT ☐

OVULATION / PREGNANCY SIGNS

TESTS / MEDS / PROCEDURES

EXERCISE

RELAXATION

NOTES

CONCEPTION WONDERS   Eggs of any species are roughly the same size—about 1/200 of an inch in diameter—though the size of the egg-containing follicle is roughly related to the size of the animal. A whale's eggs could pass through a rat's tubes, even though the whale egg's follicle could be as big as a rabbit.

Friday
__/__

CYCLE DAY ☐   PRENATAL SUPPLEMENT ☐

OVULATION / PREGNANCY SIGNS

TESTS / MEDS / PROCEDURES

EXERCISE

NOTES

RELAXATION

Saturday
__/__

CYCLE DAY ☐   PRENATAL SUPPLEMENT ☐

OVULATION / PREGNANCY SIGNS

TESTS / MEDS / PROCEDURES

EXERCISE

NOTES

RELAXATION

THROUGH THE AGES   In 1954, an Illinois court ruled that donor insemination was "contrary to good morals"—even if a husband consented to it—and was considered adultery on the mother's part. A donor-sperm child was deemed "born out of wedlock and therefore illegitimate." In 1964, Georgia became the first state to legitimize donor-sperm children.

Sunday   __/__

CYCLE DAY ☐   PRENATAL SUPPLEMENT ☐

OVULATION / PREGNANCY SIGNS

TESTS / MEDS / PROCEDURES

EXERCISE

NOTES

RELAXATION

Week in Review

GOAL CHECK _____

TOTAL EXERCISE SESSIONS _____

TOTAL RELAXATION SESSIONS_____

THOUGHTS AND FEELINGS

WEEK
20

DATES: _____

GOALS: _____
_____
_____
_____

Monday   __/__

CYCLE DAY ☐   PRENATAL SUPPLEMENT ☐

OVULATION / PREGNANCY SIGNS	TESTS / MEDS / PROCEDURES
	_____
	_____
	_____
	_____
	_____

EXERCISE

_____
_____
_____
_____

RELAXATION

_____
_____
_____
_____

NOTES

Tuesday   __/__

CYCLE DAY ☐   PRENATAL SUPPLEMENT ☐

OVULATION / PREGNANCY SIGNS	TESTS / MEDS / PROCEDURES
	_____
	_____
	_____
	_____

EXERCISE

_____
_____
_____

RELAXATION

_____
_____
_____

NOTES

BY THE NUMBERS   65 to 70: Percentage of frozen embryos that survive thaw. **30 to 35:** Percentage of frozen embryos with 100 percent cell survival. These embryos are almost as likely to implant as those never frozen. However, even thawed embryos that survive with 50 percent of their cells intact still have a decent chance of implanting.

Wednesday   __/__

CYCLE DAY ☐   PRENATAL SUPPLEMENT ☐

OVULATION / PREGNANCY SIGNS

TESTS / MEDS / PROCEDURES

_____
_____
_____
_____

EXERCISE

_____
_____
_____

NOTES

RELAXATION

_____
_____
_____
_____

Thursday   __/__

CYCLE DAY ☐   PRENATAL SUPPLEMENT ☐

OVULATION / PREGNANCY SIGNS

TESTS / MEDS / PROCEDURES

_____
_____
_____
_____

EXERCISE

_____
_____
_____

NOTES

RELAXATION

_____
_____
_____

MYTH VS. REALITY **Myth:** You can't get pregnant while breast-feeding. **Reality:** Although you may not get your period for several months after giving birth, you could start ovulating at any time and probably won't know when it happens.

Friday
___/___

CYCLE DAY ☐   PRENATAL SUPPLEMENT ☐

OVULATION / PREGNANCY SIGNS

TESTS / MEDS / PROCEDURES

EXERCISE

NOTES

RELAXATION

Saturday
___/___

CYCLE DAY ☐   PRENATAL SUPPLEMENT ☐

OVULATION / PREGNANCY SIGNS

TESTS / MEDS / PROCEDURES

EXERCISE

NOTES

RELAXATION

THROUGH THE AGES An Italian noted in 1776 that sperm cooled by snow stopped moving, but the first big breakthrough in sperm freezing came in 1949, when British scientists accidentally discovered that glycerol, a syrupy substance, could protect frozen sperm from damage. The first successful human pregnancy conceived with frozen sperm was reported four years later.

Sunday ___/___

CYCLE DAY ☐   PRENATAL SUPPLEMENT ☐

OVULATION / PREGNANCY SIGNS

TESTS / MEDS / PROCEDURES

EXERCISE

RELAXATION

NOTES

Week in Review

GOAL CHECK _____

TOTAL EXERCISE SESSIONS _____

TOTAL RELAXATION SESSIONS _____

THOUGHTS AND FEELINGS

21

DATES: _____

GOALS: _____
_____
_____
_____

Monday

—/—

CYCLE DAY ☐   PRENATAL SUPPLEMENT ☐

OVULATION / PREGNANCY SIGNS

TESTS / MEDS / PROCEDURES
_____
_____
_____
_____
_____

EXERCISE
_____
_____
_____

RELAXATION
_____
_____
_____
_____

NOTES

Tuesday

—/—

CYCLE DAY ☐   PRENATAL SUPPLEMENT ☐

OVULATION / PREGNANCY SIGNS

TESTS / MEDS / PROCEDURES
_____
_____
_____
_____
_____

EXERCISE
_____
_____
_____

RELAXATION
_____
_____
_____

NOTES

BY THE NUMBERS **1980:** Year that an eccentric California optometrist opened the so-called Nobel Prize sperm bank, ostensibly stocked with the seed of geniuses, to help save humankind from being overrun by "retrograde humans." **3:** Number of actual Nobel laureates who donated sperm. **215:** Number of children produced via the sperm bank. **0:** Number of Nobel babies produced. **1999:** Year the sperm bank closed.

Wednesday —/—

CYCLE DAY ☐   PRENATAL SUPPLEMENT ☐

OVULATION / PREGNANCY SIGNS

TESTS / MEDS / PROCEDURES

_____
_____
_____
_____
_____

EXERCISE

_____
_____
_____
_____

NOTES

RELAXATION

_____
_____
_____

Thursday —/—

CYCLE DAY ☐   PRENATAL SUPPLEMENT ☐

OVULATION / PREGNANCY SIGNS

TESTS / MEDS / PROCEDURES

_____
_____
_____
_____
_____

EXERCISE

_____
_____
_____
_____

NOTES

RELAXATION

_____
_____
_____
_____

CONCEPTION WONDERS   The world's oldest man to father a child was reportedly Australian miner Les Colley, whose Fijian wife, whom he met through a dating service, gave birth when Colley was either 92 or 93—reports differ. According to U.S. state databases, numerous American men have fathered children at ages 88 and 89.

Friday   —/—

CYCLE DAY ☐   PRENATAL SUPPLEMENT ☐

OVULATION / PREGNANCY SIGNS

TESTS / MEDS / PROCEDURES

EXERCISE

RELAXATION

NOTES

Saturday   —/—

CYCLE DAY ☐   PRENATAL SUPPLEMENT ☐

OVULATION / PREGNANCY SIGNS

TESTS / MEDS / PROCEDURES

EXERCISE

RELAXATION

NOTES

THROUGH THE AGES The first scientific pregnancy test, developed in 1928, involved injecting a woman's urine into mice. One hundred hours later, the mice were killed and their ovaries examined. A 1931 test used rabbits, reducing the wait to 48 hours. Even faster: A 1939 version used frogs, with results in 12 hours.

Sunday ___/___

| CYCLE DAY | ☐ | PRENATAL SUPPLEMENT | ☐ |

OVULATION / PREGNANCY SIGNS

TESTS / MEDS / PROCEDURES

_____
_____
_____
_____
_____

EXERCISE

_____
_____
_____
_____

RELAXATION

_____
_____
_____
_____

NOTES

Week in Review

GOAL CHECK _____

TOTAL EXERCISE SESSIONS _____

TOTAL RELAXATION SESSIONS _____

THOUGHTS AND FEELINGS

WEEK
22

DATES: _____

GOALS: _____

_____

_____

_____

Monday
___/___

CYCLE DAY ☐   PRENATAL SUPPLEMENT ☐

OVULATION / PREGNANCY SIGNS

TESTS / MEDS / PROCEDURES

_____

_____

_____

_____

_____

EXERCISE

_____

_____

_____

RELAXATION

_____

_____

_____

_____

NOTES

Tuesday
___/___

CYCLE DAY ☐   PRENATAL SUPPLEMENT ☐

OVULATION / PREGNANCY SIGNS

TESTS / MEDS / PROCEDURES

_____

_____

_____

_____

_____

EXERCISE

_____

_____

_____

RELAXATION

_____

_____

_____

_____

NOTES

BY THE NUMBERS **1983:** Birth of first baby conceived via IVF with a donor egg. **12:** Percentage of all IVFs that involve a donor egg. **51:** Approximate percentage, nationwide, of IVF transfers using fresh donor eggs that result in a live birth. **34.7:** Percent of IVF transfers using fresh nondonor eggs that result in a live birth.

Wednesday ___/___

CYCLE DAY ☐   PRENATAL SUPPLEMENT ☐

OVULATION / PREGNANCY SIGNS

TESTS / MEDS / PROCEDURES

EXERCISE

RELAXATION

NOTES

Thursday ___/___

CYCLE DAY ☐   PRENATAL SUPPLEMENT ☐

OVULATION / PREGNANCY SIGNS

TESTS / MEDS / PROCEDURES

EXERCISE

RELAXATION

NOTES

MYTH VS. REALITY **Myth:** Having sex closer to ovulation will decrease your chances of conceiving a girl. **Reality:** When you have sex—whether 5 days before you ovulate or the day of ovulation—has no influence on the sex of the baby, according to a study published in the *New England Journal of Medicine*.

Friday ___/___

CYCLE DAY ☐   PRENATAL SUPPLEMENT ☐

OVULATION / PREGNANCY SIGNS

TESTS / MEDS / PROCEDURES

_____
_____
_____
_____

EXERCISE

_____
_____
_____

RELAXATION

_____
_____
_____

NOTES

Saturday ___/___

CYCLE DAY ☐   PRENATAL SUPPLEMENT ☐

OVULATION / PREGNANCY SIGNS

TESTS / MEDS / PROCEDURES

_____
_____
_____
_____

EXERCISE

_____
_____
_____

RELAXATION

_____
_____
_____

NOTES

THROUGH THE AGES In the 1950s, some doctors would mix donor sperm with a sterile father's sperm so that the father could pretend his own boys had performed. Most patients went to one doctor for the insemination and another for the pregnancy so the doctor delivering the baby wouldn't know the father wasn't the biological father.

Sunday

__/__

CYCLE DAY ☐   PRENATAL SUPPLEMENT ☐

OVULATION / PREGNANCY SIGNS

TESTS / MEDS / PROCEDURES
_____
_____
_____
_____
_____

EXERCISE
_____
_____
_____
_____

RELAXATION
_____
_____
_____
_____

NOTES

Week in Review

GOAL CHECK _____

TOTAL EXERCISE SESSIONS _____

TOTAL RELAXATION SESSIONS _____

THOUGHTS AND FEELINGS

WEEK
23

DATES: _____

GOALS: _____

_____

_____

_____

Monday

__/__

CYCLE DAY ☐   PRENATAL SUPPLEMENT ☐

OVULATION / PREGNANCY SIGNS

TESTS / MEDS / PROCEDURES

_____

_____

_____

_____

_____

EXERCISE

_____

_____

_____

NOTES

RELAXATION

_____

_____

_____

_____

Tuesday

__/__

CYCLE DAY ☐   PRENATAL SUPPLEMENT ☐

OVULATION / PREGNANCY SIGNS

TESTS / MEDS / PROCEDURES

_____

_____

_____

_____

_____

EXERCISE

_____

_____

_____

NOTES

RELAXATION

_____

_____

_____

BY THE NUMBERS **30:** Number of minutes it takes sperm to reach the fallopian tubes once they penetrate the cervical mucus. **15 to 60:** Minutes before sperm start penetrating the tough shell surrounding the egg. **20:** Minutes it typically takes the sperm head to drill its way through the shell.

Wednesday __/__

CYCLE DAY ☐   PRENATAL SUPPLEMENT ☐

OVULATION / PREGNANCY SIGNS

TESTS / MEDS / PROCEDURES

EXERCISE

RELAXATION

NOTES

Thursday __/__

CYCLE DAY ☐   PRENATAL SUPPLEMENT ☐

OVULATION / PREGNANCY SIGNS

TESTS / MEDS / PROCEDURES

EXERCISE

RELAXATION

NOTES

CONCEPTION WONDERS In 1997, a British woman set the record for the longest recorded interval between the birth of two of her children—41 years. Liz Buttle's daughter Belinda was born on May 19, 1956, and son Joseph on November 20, 1997, when Buttle was 60. Buttle, who used a donor egg, told her fertility clinic that she was 49.

Friday ___/___

CYCLE DAY ☐   PRENATAL SUPPLEMENT ☐

OVULATION / PREGNANCY SIGNS

TESTS / MEDS / PROCEDURES

EXERCISE

RELAXATION

NOTES

Saturday ___/___

CYCLE DAY ☐   PRENATAL SUPPLEMENT ☐

OVULATION / PREGNANCY SIGNS

TESTS / MEDS / PROCEDURES

EXERCISE

RELAXATION

NOTES

THROUGH THE AGES In ancient Greece, some believed boys were more likely to be conceived during hot weather and girls during cold. A German legend held that making love during rainy weather would produce a girl, whereas sex during dry weather would produce a boy.

Sunday

__/__

CYCLE DAY ☐   PRENATAL SUPPLEMENT ☐

OVULATION / PREGNANCY SIGNS

TESTS / MEDS / PROCEDURES

EXERCISE

RELAXATION

NOTES

Week in Review

GOAL CHECK _____

TOTAL EXERCISE SESSIONS _____

TOTAL RELAXATION SESSIONS _____

THOUGHTS AND FEELINGS

WEEK
24

DATES: _____

GOALS: _____
_____
_____
_____

Monday   __/__

CYCLE DAY [ ]   PRENATAL SUPPLEMENT [ ]

OVULATION / PREGNANCY SIGNS	TESTS / MEDS / PROCEDURES
	_____
	_____
	_____
	_____
	_____

EXERCISE

_____
_____
_____

RELAXATION

_____
_____
_____

NOTES

Tuesday   __/__

CYCLE DAY [ ]   PRENATAL SUPPLEMENT [ ]

OVULATION / PREGNANCY SIGNS	TESTS / MEDS / PROCEDURES
	_____
	_____
	_____
	_____
	_____

EXERCISE

_____
_____
_____

RELAXATION

_____
_____
_____

NOTES

BY THE NUMBERS **525:** Number of sons fathered by a ruthless seventeenth-century Moroccan emperor, through his numerous concubines. **342:** Number of daughters he fathered. Neglected during childhood, his offspring apparently became a public nuisance, given to robbing and murdering slaves.

Wednesday __/__

CYCLE DAY ☐   PRENATAL SUPPLEMENT ☐

OVULATION / PREGNANCY SIGNS

TESTS / MEDS / PROCEDURES

_____
_____
_____
_____
_____

EXERCISE

_____
_____
_____

RELAXATION

_____
_____
_____

NOTES

Thursday __/__

CYCLE DAY ☐   PRENATAL SUPPLEMENT ☐

OVULATION / PREGNANCY SIGNS

TESTS / MEDS / PROCEDURES

_____
_____
_____
_____
_____

EXERCISE

_____
_____
_____

RELAXATION

_____
_____
_____

NOTES

MYTH VS. REALITY **Myth:** Abstaining from sex for a week can boost a man's sperm count. **Reality:** Although intercourse does partially deplete men of sperm, there's no benefit to abstaining for more than 4 or 5 days before a sperm count test or an attempt at conception.

Friday   __/__

CYCLE DAY ☐   PRENATAL SUPPLEMENT ☐

OVULATION / PREGNANCY SIGNS

TESTS / MEDS / PROCEDURES
_____
_____
_____
_____
_____

EXERCISE
_____
_____
_____

RELAXATION
_____
_____
_____

NOTES

Saturday   __/__

CYCLE DAY ☐   PRENATAL SUPPLEMENT ☐

OVULATION / PREGNANCY SIGNS

TESTS / MEDS / PROCEDURES
_____
_____
_____
_____

EXERCISE
_____
_____
_____

RELAXATION
_____
_____
_____

NOTES

THROUGH THE AGES   In 1944, a Harvard gynecologist took first steps toward human IVF, retrieving a woman's eggs during abdominal surgery and incubating them for 27 hours before mixing them with sperm. When he reported successful fertilization, skeptics called it "reflex cell division" that could never lead to a healthy child.

Sunday   __/__

CYCLE DAY ☐   PRENATAL SUPPLEMENT ☐

OVULATION / PREGNANCY SIGNS

TESTS / MEDS / PROCEDURES

EXERCISE

RELAXATION

NOTES

Week in Review

GOAL CHECK _____

TOTAL EXERCISE SESSIONS _____

TOTAL RELAXATION SESSIONS _____

THOUGHTS AND FEELINGS

MONTH-AT-A-GLANCE CALENDARS

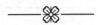

The daily log gives you plenty of space to track your cycle in detail; what a monthly calendar offers is the big picture. When it comes to detecting patterns in your cycle, both are important. On the following pages you'll find six month-at-a-glance calendars with blank spaces so that you can fill in the month and dates. You may want to transfer these (and perhaps other) key items from your daily log to your monthly calendar:

- The first day of your period
- When you think you're ovulating
- When you have sex
- When you have an IUI, egg retrieval, or IVF transfer
- Medical appointments
- Key blood test and ultrasound results
- Medications and dosages

Month ____

S	M	T	W	T	F	S
⌐	⌐	⌐	⌐	⌐	⌐	⌐
⌐	⌐	⌐	⌐	⌐	⌐	⌐
⌐	⌐	⌐	⌐	⌐	⌐	⌐
⌐	⌐	⌐	⌐	⌐	⌐	⌐
⌐	⌐	⌐	⌐	⌐	⌐	⌐

Month _____

S	M	T	W	T	F	S

Month _____

S	M	T	W	T	F	S
	└	└	└	└	└	└
└	└	└	└	└	└	└
└	└	└	└	└	└	└
└	└	└	└	└	└	└
└	└	└	└	└	└	└

Month _____

S	M	T	W	T	F	S
⌐	⌐	⌐	⌐	⌐	⌐	⌐
⌐	⌐	⌐	⌐	⌐	⌐	⌐
⌐	⌐	⌐	⌐	⌐	⌐	⌐
⌐	⌐	⌐	⌐	⌐	⌐	⌐
⌐	⌐	⌐	⌐	⌐	⌐	⌐

Month ____

S	M	T	W	T	F	S

Month _____

S	M	T	W	T	F	S
⌐	⌐	⌐	⌐	⌐	⌐	⌐
⌐	⌐	⌐	⌐	⌐	⌐	⌐
⌐	⌐	⌐	⌐	⌐	⌐	⌐
⌐	⌐	⌐	⌐	⌐	⌐	⌐
⌐	⌐	⌐	⌐	⌐	⌐	⌐

BASAL BODY TEMPERATURE (BBT) CHARTS

Although tracking your morning temperature won't help you time sex, as explained on page 23, you can use BBT charting to find out whether you ovulate. At some point during your cycle, your temperature should spike about half a degree and stay there until your next period. This isn't true for all women; a small percentage have a relatively even temperature pattern and yet still ovulate. That's why it's a good idea to use BBT charting in conjunction with the other methods described in the "Using Your Log" section. (You may find it easier to skip the charting and use the other methods instead.)

To learn everything you ever wanted to know about BBT charting, including how to deal with daylight savings time and travel to other time zones, refer to *Taking Charge of Your Fertility* (www.tcoyf.com) by Toni Weschler. Here are some basic guidelines for tracking your BBT:

- Use an oral, digital, basal body thermometer.

- Day 1 of your chart should be the first day of full menstrual flow, not spotting.
- Shake down the thermometer before going to bed, since even the act of shaking it in the morning can raise your temperature.
- Leave the thermometer by your bed. If you have to walk to the bathroom in the morning, you may inadvertently raise your temperature and skew the chart.
- Take your temperature first thing in the morning before you get out of bed or talk on the phone, at roughly the same time each day. Place the thermometer under your tongue for at least two or three minutes.
- Record your temperature by using a dot, and make this mark immediately.
- Make a note when you're sick or when you've stayed up late or slept poorly. All these things can affect your temperature.
- Start a new chart when you get your next period.

Basal Body Temperature Chart

DATES COVERED: DAY _____ MONTH _____ YEAR _____ TO DAY _____ MONTH _____ YEAR _____

CYCLE DAY	1	2	3	4	5	6	7	8	9	10	11	12	13	14	15	16	17	18	19	20	21	22	23	24	25	26	27	28	29	30	31	32	33	34	35	36
WEEKDAY																																				
DATE																																				
TIME																																				
99.1																																				
99.0																																				
98.9																																				
98.8																																				
98.7																																				
98.6																																				
98.5																																				
98.4																																				
98.3																																				
98.2																																				
98.1																																				
98.0																																				
97.9																																				
97.8																																				
97.7																																				
97.6																																				
97.5																																				
97.4																																				
97.3																																				
97.2																																				
97.1																																				
97.0																																				
96.9																																				

Notes: (List any changes to your routine)

Basal Body Temperature Chart

DATES COVERED: DAY ____ MONTH ____ YEAR ____ TO DAY ____ MONTH ____ YEAR ____

CYCLE DAY	1	2	3	4	5	6	7	8	9	10	11	12	13	14	15	16	17	18	19	20	21	22	23	24	25	26	27	28	29	30	31	32	33	34	35	36
WEEKDAY																																				
DATE																																				
TIME																																				
99.1																																				
99.0																																				
98.9																																				
98.8																																				
98.7																																				
98.6																																				
98.5																																				
98.4																																				
98.3																																				
98.2																																				
98.1																																				
98.0																																				
97.9																																				
97.8																																				
97.7																																				
97.6																																				
97.5																																				
97.4																																				
97.3																																				
97.2																																				
97.1																																				
97.0																																				
96.9																																				

Notes: (List any changes to your routine)

Basal Body Temperature Chart

DATES COVERED: DAY____ MONTH____ YEAR____ TO DAY____ MONTH____ YEAR____

CYCLE DAY	1	2	3	4	5	6	7	8	9	10	11	12	13	14	15	16	17	18	19	20	21	22	23	24	25	26	27	28	29	30	31	32	33	34	35	36
WEEKDAY																																				
DATE																																				
TIME																																				
99.1																																				
99.0																																				
98.9																																				
98.8																																				
98.7																																				
98.6																																				
98.5																																				
98.4																																				
98.3																																				
98.2																																				
98.1																																				
98.0																																				
97.9																																				
97.8																																				
97.7																																				
97.6																																				
97.5																																				
97.4																																				
97.3																																				
97.2																																				
97.1																																				
97.0																																				
96.9																																				

Notes: (List any changes to your routine)

Basal Body Temperature Chart

DATES COVERED: DAY ____ MONTH ____ YEAR ____ TO DAY ____ MONTH ____ YEAR ____

CYCLE DAY	1	2	3	4	5	6	7	8	9	10	11	12	13	14	15	16	17	18	19	20	21	22	23	24	25	26	27	28	29	30	31	32	33	34	35	36
WEEKDAY																																				
DATE																																				
TIME																																				
99.1																																				
99.0																																				
98.9																																				
98.8																																				
98.7																																				
98.6																																				
98.5																																				
98.4																																				
98.3																																				
98.2																																				
98.1																																				
98.0																																				
97.9																																				
97.8																																				
97.7																																				
97.6																																				
97.5																																				
97.4																																				
97.3																																				
97.2																																				
97.1																																				
97.0																																				
96.9																																				

Notes: (List any changes to your routine)

Basal Body Temperature Chart

DATES COVERED: DAY ____ MONTH ____ YEAR ____ TO DAY ____ MONTH ____ YEAR ____

CYCLE DAY	1	2	3	4	5	6	7	8	9	10	11	12	13	14	15	16	17	18	19	20	21	22	23	24	25	26	27	28	29	30	31	32	33	34	35	36
WEEKDAY																																				
DATE																																				
TIME																																				
99.1																																				
99.0																																				
98.9																																				
98.8																																				
98.7																																				
98.6																																				
98.5																																				
98.4																																				
98.3																																				
98.2																																				
98.1																																				
98.0																																				
97.9																																				
97.8																																				
97.7																																				
97.6																																				
97.5																																				
97.4																																				
97.3																																				
97.2																																				
97.1																																				
97.0																																				
96.9																																				

Notes: (List any changes to your routine)

Basal Body Temperature Chart

DATES COVERED: DAY ____ MONTH ____ YEAR ____ TO DAY ____ MONTH ____ YEAR ____

CYCLE DAY	1	2	3	4	5	6	7	8	9	10	11	12	13	14	15	16	17	18	19	20	21	22	23	24	25	26	27	28	29	30	31	32	33	34	35	36
WEEKDAY																																				
DATE																																				
TIME																																				
99.1																																				
99.0																																				
98.9																																				
98.8																																				
98.7																																				
98.6																																				
98.5																																				
98.4																																				
98.3																																				
98.2																																				
98.1																																				
98.0																																				
97.9																																				
97.8																																				
97.7																																				
97.6																																				
97.5																																				
97.4																																				
97.3																																				
97.2																																				
97.1																																				
97.0																																				
96.9																																				

Notes: (List any changes to your routine)

TEST RESULTS

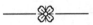

My Test Results

DATE	TEST	RESULTS

My Partner's Test Results

DATE	TEST	RESULTS

FOUR-DAY
JOURNALING EXERCISE

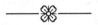

If you've had your share of disappointments on the fertility front, give journal writing a try. It's a coping strategy commonly used in mind/body infertility programs, and research suggests that it is quite effective. "Infertility treatments are often associated with great stress as well as secrecy," says James Pennebaker, chair of the psychology department at the University of Texas, Austin, and a leading researcher on the health benefits of expressive writing. "People are dealing with major issues in their lives that are difficult to talk about with friends and family. There is some evidence that writing works particularly well for people who aren't able to openly discuss troubling topics with others."

In many mind/body infertility programs, participants are given a four-day journaling exercise as homework. "We instruct them to write about the most distressing part of the infertility experience—what's really been a trauma for them," says Leslee Kagan of the Harvard Mind/Body Medical Institute. The trauma could be a failed IVF or a miscarriage or the deterioration of a relationship with a fertile sister or friend. Often, Kagan says, writing about this ordeal helps women discover insights buried deep within them that become integral to the healing process.

"The ultimate skill in coping is to make some meaning out of a trauma," Kagan says. For example, through journaling many women recognize how close they've become to their husbands. Though they'd never have wished this experience on themselves, it has taken them to a level of intimacy they might not have otherwise achieved. "Creating an awareness of some way in which this experience has changed them—an appreciation of this different route they traveled—is a very freeing experience," Kagan notes.

Following are rough guidelines for a journaling exercise, adapted from Pennebaker's research. "Keep in mind that there are probably a thousand ways to write that may be beneficial to you," Pennebaker says. Experiment and see what works best for you.

- Commit to writing for at least fifteen minutes a day for at least four consecutive days.
- Find a time and place where you won't be disturbed. Ideally, write at the end of your workday or before you go to bed.
- Once you begin writing, write continuously. Don't worry about spelling or grammar—nobody will ever read this! If you run out of things to write about, just repeat what you have already written.
- You can write about the same topic on all four days, or write about something different each day. It's your decision.
- Experiment with different formats. For example, if "Dear diary" style seems too contrived, try writing a letter to a

particular person—your husband, a friend, your doctor—or craft a speech or a dialogue with someone else.

- Write on a computer rather than in this journal if you prefer. To keep all your fertility-related materials in one place, you may want to print out your journal and staple it into the back pages of this log.

Date _____

Date _____

Date _____

Date _____

Date _____

Date _____

Date _____

Date _____

Date _____

Date _____

RECOMMENDED BOOKS AND WEB SITES

BOOKS

The Conception Chronicles: The Uncensored Truth About Sex, Love & Marriage When You're Trying to Get Pregnant, by Patty Doyle Debano, Courtney Menzel, and Shelly Sutphen.

Conquering Infertility, by Alice D. Domar and Alice Lesch Kelly.

The Couple's Guide to In Vitro Fertilization, by Liza Charlesworth.

Having Your Baby Through Egg Donation, by Ellen Sarasohn Glazer and Evelina Weidman Sterling.

How to Get Pregnant: The Classic Guide to Overcoming Infertility, by Sherman J. Silber.

The Mother of All Pregnancy Books: The Ultimate Guide to Conception, Birth, and Everything In Between, by Ann Douglas.

Overcoming Infertility: A Cleveland Clinic Guide, by Tomasso Falcone and Davis Young.

Resolving Infertility, by the staff of RESOLVE, with Diane Aronson.

Taking Charge of Your Fertility: The Definitive Guide to Natural Birth Control and Pregnancy Achievement, by Toni Weschler.

WEB SITES

A Little Pregnant, *www.alittlepregnant.com:* The best of the infertility blogs, subtitled Madcap Misadventures in Infertility, Pregnancy and Parenthood.

American College of Obstetricians and Gynecologists, *www.acog.com:* Features a physician locator by city.

American Fertility Association, *www.theafa.org:* Referrals for fertility specialists, support groups, and therapists.

American Society for Reproductive Medicine, *www.asrm.org:* Fertility FAQs and booklets, medical journal highlights, state infertility insurance laws.

BabyCenter, *www.babycenter.com/magazine:* Preconception section includes bulletin boards, chats, and articles on fertility issues, exercise, nutrition, finances.

Centers for Disease Control and Prevention, *http://www.cdc.gov/ART/ART2003/index.htm:* Yearly reports on Assisted Reproductive Technology success rates for clinics in the United States.

Conceive Magazine, *www.conceivemagazine.com:* Subscription information and selected articles about conception, fertility, and adoption.

Fertility Lifelines, *www.fertilitylifelines.com:* Educational site sponsored by Sorono, manufacturer of fertility drugs.

Infertility Awareness Association of Canada, *www.iaac.ca:* Support groups, information, online chats, therapist referrals.

InterNational Council on Infertility Information Dissemination, *www.inciid.org:* Information, support, therapist and physician referrals.

RESOLVE: The National Infertility Association, *www.Resolve.org:* information, bulletin boards, chat rooms, clinical trials listings.

Society for Assisted Reproductive Technology, *www.sart.org:* ART success rates for 350+ clinics nationwide, ART patient handbook, financial information.

Taking Charge of Your Fertility, *www.tcoyf.com:* Cycle-tracking software that serves as a companion to Toni Weschler's book.

SOURCES

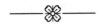

INTRODUCTION

Koen Demyttenaere et al., "Coping Style and Depression Level Influence Outcome in In Vitro Fertilization," *Fertility and Sterility* 60 (June 1998): 1026–1033.

Alice Domar et al., "The Impact of Group Psychological Interventions on Pregnancy Rates in Infertile Women," *Fertility and Sterility* 74 (April 2000): 805–811.

Alice Domar et al., "The Impact of Group Psychological Interventions on Distress in Infertile Women," *Health Psychology* 19 (November 2000): 568–575.

Robert A. Emmons and Michael McCullough, "Counting Blessings Versus Burdens: An Experimental Investigation of Gratitude and Subjective Well-Being in Daily Life," *Journal of Personal Social Psychology* 84 (February 2003): 377–389.

James W. Pennebaker, *Writing to Heal: A Guided Journal for Recovering from Trauma and Emotional Upheaval* (Oakland, CA: New Harbinger Press, 2004).

SETTING SIX-MONTH GOALS

James F. Clapp III, *Exercising Through Your Pregnancy* (Champaign, IL: Human Kinetics, 1998), 82–83.

James F. Clapp III, "Exercise During Pregnancy: A Clinical Update," *Clinical Sports Medicine* 19 (April 2000): 273–286.

DAILY JOURNAL

Week 1

BY THE NUMBERS

Sherman J. Silber, *How to Get Pregnant* (New York: Little, Brown, 2005), 53.

CONCEPTION WONDERS

1. Catherine Billey, "Identical Quadruplets Born," *New York Times*, March 27, 2002.
2. Michael B. Miller, "Multiple Birth Watch," *Twin Research* 1, no. 3 (1998), http://taxa.epi.umn.edu/twinnews/twin_1_3.htm.

THROUGH THE AGES

Clara Pinto-Correia, *The Ovary of Eve: Egg and Sperm and Preformation* (Chicago: University Of Chicago Press, 1998).

Week 2

BY THE NUMBERS

1. Joyce A. Martin et al., "Births: Final Data for 2003," *National Vital Statistics Reports* 54 (September 8, 2005), http://www.cdc.gov/nchs/data/nvsr/nvsr54/nvsr54_02.pdf.
2. "Births," *Statistics Canada* (April 19, 2004, 2002), http://www.statcan.ca/Daily/English/040419/d040419b.htm.
3. Guy Desplanques, "Population of France," Embassy of France in the United States, http://www.ambafrance-us.org/atoz/pop_fr.asp.
4. Zenit News Services, "Coming Boom Won't Be of Babies," December 20, 2003, http://www.zenit.org/english/visualizza.phtml?sid=46539.

MYTH VS. REALITY

Sherman J. Silber, *How to Get Pregnant* (New York: Little, Brown, 2005), 70.

THROUGH THE AGES
Office of NIH History, "A Thin Blue Line: History of the Home Pregnancy Test," http://history.nih.gov/exhibits/thinblueline/research4.html.

Week 3

BY THE NUMBERS
1. Sonia Fader, "Sperm Banking: A Reproductive Resource," California Cryobank, 1993, *cryobank.com*, http://www.cryobank.com/sbanking.cfm?page=2&sub=126.
2. Associated Press, "First Baby Born of Frozen Embryo," April 11, 1984.
3. Shari Roan, "Infertility Researchers Find Success Using Frozen Eggs," *Los Angeles Times*, October 17, 1997, 2.
4. BBC News, "First 'Frozen' Twins Born," December 29, 2000, http://news.bbc.co.uk/1/hi/health/1092079.stm.
5. "Nurse Delivers World's First Baby from Frozen Donor Egg," *ScienceDaily.com*, January 4, 2006, http://www.sciencedaily.com/releases/2006/01/060103184649.htm.

CONCEPTION WONDERS
Sherman J. Silber, *How to Get Pregnant* (New York: Little, Brown, 2005), xxix.

THROUGH THE AGES
Office of NIH History, "A Thin Blue Line: History of the Home Pregnancy Test," http://history.nih.gov/exhibits/thinblueline/timeline.html.

Week 4

BY THE NUMBERS
Sherman J. Silber, *How to Get Pregnant* (New York: Little, Brown, 2005), 87.

THROUGH THE AGES

Gena Corea, *The Mother Machine: Reproductive Technologies from Artificial Insemination to Artificial Wombs* (New York: Harper and Row, 1979), 12.

Week 5

BY THE NUMBERS

Sherman J. Silber, *How to Get Pregnant* (New York: Little, Brown, 2005), 6, 140.

CONCEPTION WONDERS

Shaoni Bhattacharya, "Baby Born from Sperm Frozen for 21 Years," *NewScientist.com*, May 25, 2004, http://www.newscientist.com/article.ns?id=dn5031.

THROUGH THE AGES

Robin Marantz Henig, *Pandora's Baby: How the First Test Tube Babies Sparked the Reproductive Revolution* (Boston: Houghton Mifflin, 2004), 50.

Week 6

BY THE NUMBERS

1. Joyce A. Martin et al., "Births: Final Data for 2003," *National Vital Statistics Reports* 54 (September 8, 2005), http://www.cdc.gov/nchs/data/nvsr/nvsr54/nvsr54_02.pdf.
2. Health Systems Trust, "SA Has Lowest Fertility Rate on African Continent," September 21, 2005, http://www.hst.org.za/news/20000913.
3. UN Wire, "Spain: Birth Rate Falls Dramatically," March 1, 2000.

MYTH VS. REALITY

Robert Munkelwitz and Bruce Gilbert, "Are Boxer Shorts Really Better? A Critical Analysis of the Role of Underwear Type in Male Subfertility," *Journal of Urology* 160 (October 1998): 1329–1333.

THROUGH THE AGES

1. Stephen Smith, "The Fertility Race: From Barren to Infertile," *American RadioWorks*, September 1999, http://americanradioworks .publicradio.org/features/fertility_race/part1/timeline.shtml.
2. "Beyond Barren: Perceptions of Female Infertility Through Time," *InfertilityCentral.com*, http://www.infertilitycentral.com/fertility/ beyond-barren-perceptions-of-female-infertility-through-time,3.html.

Week 7

BY THE NUMBERS

World Sexual Records "Conception and Prevention," *sexualrecords .com*, http://www.sexualrecords.com/WSRprev.html.

CONCEPTION WONDERS

1. R. E. Wenk et al., "How Frequent Is Heteropaternal Superfecundation?" *Acta geneticae medicae et gemellologiae* 41, no. 1 (1992): 43–47.
2. E. Girela et al., "Indisputable Double Paternity in Dizygous Twins," *Fertility and Sterility* 67, no. 6 (1997): 1159–1161.

THROUGH THE AGES

Robin Elise Weiss, "The Rabbit Died," Your Guide to Pregnancy/ Birth, about.com, http://pregnancy.about.com/cs/pregnancytests/a/ rabbittest.htm.

Week 8

BY THE NUMBERS

1. Vincent Iannelli, "Twin Statistics," *keepkidshealthy.com*, http:// www.keepkidshealthy.com/twins/twin_statistics.html.
2. Wikipedia, "Twin," *wikipedia.org*, http://en.wikipedia.org/wiki/Twin.

THROUGH THE AGES

Yana Mikheeva, "Boy or Girl?" *ezinearticles.com*, http://www.ezine articles.com/?Boy-or-Girl?&id=173532.

Week 9

CONCEPTION WONDERS

Carey Goldberg, "Parenthood: How Old Is Too Old?" *Boston Globe*, April 5, 2005, http://www.boston.com/news/globe/health_science/ articles/2005/04/05/parentohood_how_old_is_too_old?mode=PF.

"Woman Is Oldest Twins Mum at 59," http://www.news.bbc.co.uk/2/hi/ health/5144208.stm.

THROUGH THE AGES

David Plotz, *The Genius Factory* (New York: Random House, 2005), 161.

Week 10

BY THE NUMBERS

Sherman J. Silber, *How to Get Pregnant* (New York: Little, Brown, 2005), 31.

THROUGH THE AGES

David Plotz, *The Genius Factory* (New York: Random House, 2005), 171.

Week 11

BY THE NUMBERS

Vincent Iannelli, "Facts About Twins," *keepkidshealthy.com*, http:// www.keepkidshealthy.com/twins/expecting_twins.html.

CONCEPTION WONDERS

F. I. Seymour, C. Duffy, and C. A. Korner, "A Case of Authentic Fertility in a Man of 94," *Journal of the American Medical Association* 105 (1935): 1423–1424.

THROUGH THE AGES

Robin Marantz Henig, *Pandora's Baby: How the First Test Tube Babies Sparked the Reproductive Revolution* (Boston: Houghton Mifflin, 2004), 192, 203, 227.

Week 12

BY THE NUMBERS
Sherman J. Silber, *How to Get Pregnant* (New York: Little, Brown, 2005), 87.

THROUGH THE AGES
Sherman J. Silber, *How to Get Pregnant* (New York: Little, Brown, 2005), 32–33.

Week 13

BY THE NUMBERS
Sherman J. Silber, *How to Get Pregnant* (New York: Little, Brown, 2005), 140–141, 153.

CONCEPTION WONDERS
Rick Weiss, "Birth of Child Called First from Frozen Ovarian Tissue," *Washington Post*, September 24, 2004, A1.

THROUGH THE AGES
David Plotz, The Genius Factory (New York: Random House, 2005), 168.

Week 14

BY THE NUMBERS
U.S Census Bureau, "Record Share of New Mothers in Labor Force Census Bureau Reports," United States Department of Commerce News, October 24, 2000, http://www.census.gov/Press-Release/www/2000/cb00-175.html.

MYTH VS. REALITY
Sherman J. Silber, *How to Get Pregnant* (New York: Little, Brown, 2005), 33.

THROUGH THE AGES

Gena Corea, *The Mother Machine: Reproductive Technologies from Artificial Insemination to Artificial Wombs* (New York: Harper and Row, 1979), 40.

Week 15

BY THE NUMBERS

M. S. Neal et al., "Sidestream Smoking Is Equally As Damaging As Mainstream Smoking on IVF Outcomes," *Human Reproduction* 20 (September 2005): 2531–255.

CONCEPTION WONDERS

1. Guinness World Records, "Shortest Interval Between Separate Births Shortest Interval Between Separate Births," *Human Body/ Medical Marvels*, *guinnessworldrecords.com*, http://www.guinness worldrecords.com/content_pages/record.asp?recordid=48344.
2. "Close-Up Siblings One for the Book," *New Zealand Herald*, December 20, 2001.

THROUGH THE AGES

Alison Thiele, "Ancient Egyptian Midwifery and Childbirth," EMuseum at Minnesota State University, Manketo, http://www.mnsu.edu/ emuseum/prehistory/egypt/dailylife/midwifery.htm.

Week 16

BY THE NUMBERS

Gary Steinman, "Mechanisms of Twinning: Effect of Diet and Heredity on Twinning Rate," *Journal of Reproductive Medicine* (May 2006): 405–410.

THROUGH THE AGES

Winnie Allingham, "What Is Sperm?" *The Sex Files*, episode 3, Discovery Channel, *discoverychannel.ca*, http://discoverychannel.ca/sex files/season_1/sfs103c1.shtml.

Week 17

BY THE NUMBERS

Winnie Allingham, "What Is Sperm?" *The Sex Files*, episode 3, Discovery Channel, *discoverychannel.ca*, http://discoverychannel.ca/sex files/season_1/sfs103c1.shtml.

CONCEPTION WONDERS

"Facts & Figures: Famous Twins and Much More," *twinsworld.com*, http://www.twinsworld.com/stats.html.

THROUGH THE AGES

Office of NIH History, "A Thin Blue Line: History of the Home Pregnancy Test," http://history.nih.gov/exhibits/thinblueline/timeline.html.

Week 18

MYTH VS. REALITY

Bruce Flamm, "Ask the Experts," *babycenter.com*, http://www.babycenter.com/expert/preconception/gettingpregnant/1334780.html?ccRelLink=&url=%2Frefcap%2F3195.html&xTopic=boostchances&bus=content.

THROUGH THE AGES

Robin Marantz Henig, *Pandora's Baby: How the First Test Tube Babies Sparked the Reproductive Revolution* (Boston: Houghton Mifflin, 2004).

Week 19

BY THE NUMBERS

Pamela Prindle Fiero, "Increase or Decrease Your Chances of Having Twins/Multiples," April 14, 2006, *about.com*, http://multiples.about.com/cs/funfacts/a/oddsoftwins_2.htm.

CONCEPTION WONDERS
Sherman J. Silber, *How to Get Pregnant* (New York: Little, Brown, 2005), 21.

THROUGH THE AGES
Gena Corea, *The Mother Machine: Reproductive Technologies from Artificial Insemination to Artificial Wombs* (New York: Harper and Row, 1979), 40.

Week 20

BY THE NUMBERS
Genetics and IVF Institute, "Embryo Cropreservation," *givf.com*, http://www.givf.com/embryov.cfm.

THROUGH THE AGES
Sonia Fader, "Sperm Banking: A Reproductive Resource," California Cryobank, 1993, *cryobank.com*, http://www.cryobank.com/sbanking .cfm?page=2&sub=126.

Week 21

BY THE NUMBERS
David Plotz, *The Genius Factory* (New York: Random House, 2005), 161.

CONCEPTION WONDERS
1. "Who's Broody Now?" *Guardian Unlimited*, May 3, 2006, *guardian .co.uk*, http://www.guardian.co.uk/science/story/0,,1766358,00.html.
2. "Contest: Who Is the World's Oldest Living Father?" Gerontology Research Group, June 23, 2002, *grg.org*, http://www.grg.org/breaking news2002.htm.

THROUGH THE AGES
German Inventions and Discoveries, *german.about.com*, http://german .about.com/library/blfroschtest.htm.

Week 22

BY THE NUMBERS

2003 Assisted Reproductive Technology (ART) Report, sec. 2, "ART Cycles Using Fresh, Nondonor Eggs or Embryos," and sec. 4, "ART Cycles Using Donor Eggs," Centers for Disease Control and Prevention, http://www.cdc.gov/ART/ART2003/index.htm.

MYTH VS. REALITY

Allen J. Wilcox, Clarice R. Weinberg, and Donna D. Baird, "Timing of Sexual Intercourse in Relation to Ovulation—Effects on the Probability of Conception, Survival of the Pregnancy, and Sex of the Baby," *New England Journal of Medicine* 333 (December 7, 1995): 1517–1521.

THROUGH THE AGES.

David Plotz, *The Genius Factory* (New York: Random House, 2005), 165.

Week 23

BY THE NUMBERS

Sherman J. Silber, *How to Get Pregnant* (New York: Little, Brown, 2005), 8, 23.

CONCEPTION WONDERS

1. Reuters, "Britain's Oldest Mother at 60," *Deccan Herald*, May 5, 2006, *deccanherald.com*, http://www.deccanherald.com/deccan herald/May52006/foreign163225200654.asp.
2. Guinness World Records, *Human Body/Medical Marvels*, *guinness worldrecords.com*, http://www.guinnessworldrecords.com/index/ records.asp?id=6&pg=1.

THROUGH THE AGES

Yana Mikheeva, "Boy or Girl?" *ezinearticles.com*, http://www.ezinearticles .com/?Boy-or-Girl?&id=173532.

Week 24

MYTH VS. REALITY

Sherman J. Silber, *How to Get Pregnant* (New York: Little, Brown, 2005), 151.

THROUGH THE AGES

Robin Marantz Henig, *Pandora's Baby: How the First Test Tube Babies Sparked the Reproductive Revolution* (Boston: Houghton Mifflin Company, 2004), 30.

ACKNOWLEDGMENTS

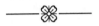

I'm so grateful to my editor, Marnie Cochran, for encouraging me to propose this book. Your enthusiasm made all the difference.

I'm also indebted to Sarah Bowen Shea and Alice Kelly, as well as Liz Neporent and Nancy Gottesman, for pointing me in the right direction when I veered off course. I'm lucky to have friends who tell it like it is.

I'm also lucky to have a husband who's not only the best shot-giver but also a stellar computer guy. Thank you, Paul, for all your help on the designs and for putting up with your squeamish wife. And muchas gracias, John Kearney, for a fabulous job filling in as my Injector.

A special thanks to Naree Viner for testing out the log format and offering thoughtful suggestions.

The staff at the Portland Center for Reproductive Medicine has been nothing but kind and professional throughout this process. I'm especially thankful to Dr. John Hesla and Andrea Speck-Zulack for taking the time to review this manuscript.